DIETARY SUPPLEMENTS: PRIMER AND FDA OVERSIGHT

NUTRITION AND DIET RESEARCH PROGRESS SERIES

Diet Quality of Americans
Nancy Cole and Mary Kay Fox
2009. ISBN: 978-1-60692-777-9 (Hardcover Book)

Diet Quality of Americans
Nancy Cole and Mary Kay Fox
2009. ISBN: 978-1-60876-499-0 (Online Book)

School Nutrition and Children
Thomas J. Baxter
2009. ISBN: 978-1-60692-891-2

Appetite and Nutritional Assessment
Shane J. Ellsworth and Reece C. Schuster (Editors)
2009. ISBN: 978-1-60741-085-0

**Flavonoids: Biosynthesis,
Biological Effects and Dietary Sources**
Raymond B. Keller (Editor)
2009. ISBN: 978-1-60741-622-7

Beta Carotene: Dietary Sources, Cancer and Cognition
Leiv Haugen and Terje Bjornson (Editors)
2009. ISBN: 978-1-60741-611-1

**Handbook of Vitamin C Research: Daily Requirements,
Dietary Sources and Adverse Effects**
Hubert Kucharski and Julek Zajac (Editors)
2009. ISBN: 978-1-60741-874-0

Dietary Supplements: Primer and FDA Oversight
Timothy H. Riley (Editor)
2010. ISBN: 978-1-60741-891-7

NUTRITION AND DIET RESEARCH PROGRESS SERIES

DIETARY SUPPLEMENTS: PRIMER AND FDA OVERSIGHT

Timothy H. Riley
Editor

Nova Science Publishers, Inc.
New York

For permission to use material from this book please contact us:
Telephone 631-231-7269; Fax 631-231-8175
Web Site: http://www.novapublishers.com

NOTICE TO THE READER

The Publisher has taken reasonable care in the preparation of this book, but makes no expressed or implied warranty of any kind and assumes no responsibility for any errors or omissions. No liability is assumed for incidental or consequential damages in connection with or arising out of information contained in this book. The Publisher shall not be liable for any special, consequential, or exemplary damages resulting, in whole or in part, from the readers' use of, or reliance upon, this material. Any parts of this book based on government reports are so indicated and copyright is claimed for those parts to the extent applicable to compilations of such works.

Independent verification should be sought for any data, advice or recommendations contained in this book. In addition, no responsibility is assumed by the publisher for any injury and/or damage to persons or property arising from any methods, products, instructions, ideas or otherwise contained in this publication.

This publication is designed to provide accurate and authoritative information with regard to the subject matter covered herein. It is sold with the clear understanding that the Publisher is not engaged in rendering legal or any other professional services. If legal or any other expert assistance is required, the services of a competent person should be sought. FROM A DECLARATION OF PARTICIPANTS JOINTLY ADOPTED BY A COMMITTEE OF THE AMERICAN BAR ASSOCIATION AND A COMMITTEE OF PUBLISHERS.

LIBRARY OF CONGRESS CATALOGING-IN-PUBLICATION DATA
    Dietary supplements : primer and FDA oversight / editor, Timothy H. Riley.
        p. ; cm.
    Includes bibliographical references and index.
    ISBN 978-1-60741-891-7 (hardcover)
    1. Dietary supplements. 2. Dietary supplements--Government policy--United States. I. Riley, Timothy H.
    [DNLM: 1. United States. Food and Drug Administration. 2. Dietary Supplements--adverse effects. 3. Government Regulation. 4. Product Surveillance, Postmarketing. 5. United States Government Agencies. QU 145.5 D5647 2009]
    RM258.5.D5445 2009
    615'.1--dc22
                                                                        2009035601

Published by Nova Science Publishers, Inc, ✦ *New York*

TABLE OF CONTENTS

PREFACE

FDA has taken some steps to identify and act upon safety concerns related to dietary supplements; however, several factors limit the agency's ability to detect concerns and remove products from the market. For example, FDA has limited information on the number and location of dietary supplement firms, the types of products currently available in the marketplace, and information about moderate and mild adverse events reported to industry. Additionally, FDA dedicates relatively few resources to oversight activities, such as providing guidance to industry regarding notification requirements for products containing new dietary ingredients. This book highlights the limited steps taken by the FDA to educate consumers about dietary supplements and their risks.This book consists of public documents which have been located, gathered, combined, reformatted, and enhanced with a subject index, selectively edited and bound to provide easy access.

Chapter 1 - Dietary supplements are substances you might use to add nutrients to your diet or to lower your risk of health problems, like osteoporosis or arthritis. Dietary supplements come in the form of pills, capsules, powders, gel tabs, extracts, or liquids. They might contain vitamins, minerals, fiber, amino acids, herbs or other plants, or enzymes. Sometimes, the ingredients in dietary supplements are added to foods, including drinks. A doctor's prescription is not needed to buy dietary supplements.

Chapter 2 - Dietary supplements and foods with added dietary ingredients, such as vitamins and herbs, constitute multibillion dollar industries. Past reports on the Food and Drug Administration's (FDA) regulation of these products raised concerns about product safety and the availability of reliable information. Since then, FDA published draft guidance on requirements for reporting adverse events—which are harmful effects or illnesses—and Current Good Manufacturing

Practice regulations for dietary supplements. GAO was asked to examine FDA's (1) actions to respond to the new serious adverse event reporting requirements, (2) ability to identify and act on concerns about the safety of dietary supplements, (3) ability to identify and act on concerns about the safety of foods with added dietary ingredients, and (4) actions to ensure that consumers have useful information about the safety and efficacy of supplements.

Chapter 3 - The law defines dietary supplements in part as products taken by mouth that contain a "dietary ingredient." Dietary ingredients include vitamins, minerals, amino acids, and herbs or botanicals, as well as other substances that can be used to supplement the diet.

Dietary supplements come in many forms, including tablets, capsules, powders, energy bars, and liquids. These products are available in stores throughout the United States, as well as on the Internet. They are labeled as dietary supplements and include among others

Chapter 4 - Some dietary supplements are beneficial when taken appropriately. Calcium supplements may strengthen bones and folic acid lowers the risk of certain birth defects. But some supplements pose health risks. They may contain harmful ingredients or be improperly manufactured or handled.

On June 22, 2007, FDA announced a final rule establishing current good manufacturing practice requirements (CGMPs) for dietary supplements. In addition, by the end of the year, industry will be required to report all serious dietary supplement adverse events to FDA.

Chapter 5 - Vitamins are essential nutrients that contribute to a healthy life. Although most people get all the vitamins they need from the foods they eat, millions of people worldwide take supplemental vitamins as part of their health regimen.

Chapter 6 - Many people take dietary supplements in an effort to be well and stay healthy. With so many dietary supplements available and so many claims made about their health benefits, how can a consumer decide what's safe and effective? This fact sheet provides a general overview of dietary supplements, discusses safety considerations, and suggests sources for additional information.

In: Dietary Supplements: Primer and FDA...   ISBN: 978-1-60741-891-7
Editors: Timothy H. Riley   © 2010 Nova Science Publishers, Inc.

Chapter 1

AGING & DIETARY SUPPLEMENTS

National Institute on Aging

DIETARY SUPPLEMENTS

Bill's retired and lives alone. Often he's just not hungry or is too tired to fix a whole meal. Does he need a multivitamin, or should he take one of those dietary supplements he sees in ads everywhere? Bill wonders if they work— will one help keep his joints healthy or another give him more energy? And, are they safe?

What Is a Dietary Supplement?

Dietary supplements are substances you might use to add nutrients to your diet or to lower your risk of health problems, like osteoporosis or arthritis. Dietary supplements come in the form of pills, capsules, powders, gel tabs, extracts, or liquids. They might contain vitamins, minerals, fiber, amino acids, herbs or other plants, or enzymes. Sometimes, the ingredients in dietary supplements are added to foods, including drinks. A doctor's prescription is not needed to buy dietary supplements.

Should I Take a Dietary Supplement?

Do you need one? Maybe you do, but usually not. Ask yourself why you think you might want to take a dietary supple-ment. Are you concerned about getting enough nutrients? Is a friend, a neighbor, or someone on a commercial suggest-ing you take one? Some ads for dietary supplements in magazines or on TV seem to promise that these supplements will make you feel better, keep you from getting sick, or even help you live longer. Sometimes, there is little, if any, good scientific research supporting these claims. Some dietary supplements will give you nutrients that might be missing from your daily diet. But eating healthy foods is the best way to get the nutrients you need. Others may cost a lot or might not benefit you the way you would like. Some supplements can change how medicines you may already be taking will work. You should talk to your doctor or a registered dietitian for advice.

What If I'm Over 50?

Peopleover50needmoreofsomevitamins and minerals than younger adults do. Your doctor or a dietitian can tell you whether you need to change your diet or take vitamins or minerals to get enough of these:

- **Vitamin B_{12}.** Vitamin B_{12} helps keep your red blood cells and nerves healthy. As people grow older, some have trouble absorbing vitamin B_{12} naturally found in food. Instead, they can choose foods, like fortified cereals, that have this vitamin added or use a B_{12} supplement.

- **Calcium.** Calcium works with vitamin D to keep bones strong at all ages. Bone loss can lead to fractures in both older women and men. Calcium is found in milk and milk products (fat-free or low-fat is best), canned fish with soft bones, dark-green leafy vegetables like spinach, and foods with calcium added.

- **Vitamin D.** Some people's bodies make enough vitamin D if they are in the sun for 10 to 15 minutes at least twice a week. But, if you are older, you may not be able to get enough vitamin D that way. Try adding vitamin D-fortified milk and milk products, vitamin D-fortified cereals, and fatty fish to your diet, and/or use a vitamin D supplement.

- **Vitamin B$_6$.** This vitamin is needed to form red blood cells. It is found in potatoes, bananas, chicken breasts, and fortified cereals.

Different Vitamin and Mineral Recommendations for People Over 50

The National Academy of Sciences recommends how much of each vitamin and mineral men and women of different ages need. Sometimes, the Academy also tells us how much of a vitamin or mineral is too much.

Vitamin B$_{12}$—2.4 mcg (micrograms) each day (if you are taking medicine for acid reflux, you might need a different form, which your health care provider can give you)

Calcium—1200 mg (milligrams), but not more than 2500 mg a day

Vitamin D—400 IU (International Units) for people age 51 to 70 and 600 IU for those over 70, but not more than 2000 IU each day

Vitamin B$_6$—1.7 mg for men and 1.5 mg for women each day

When thinking about whether you need more of a vitamin or mineral, think about how much of each nutrient you get from food and drinks, as well as from any supplements you take. Check with a doctor or dietitian to learn whether you need to supplement your diet.

What Are Antioxidants?

You might hear about *antioxidants* in the news. These are natural substances found in food that might help protect you from some diseases. Here are some common sources of antioxidants that you should be sure to include in your diet:

- *beta-carotene*—fruits and vegetables that are either dark green or dark orange
- *selenium*—seafood, liver, meat, and grains
- *vitamin C*—citrus fruits, peppers, tomatoes, and berries
- *vitamin E*—wheat germ, nuts, sesame seeds, and canola, olive, and peanut oils

Right now, research results suggest that large doses of supplements with antioxidants will not prevent chronic diseases such as heart disease or diabetes. In fact, some studies have shown that taking large doses of some antioxidants could be harmful. Again, it is best to check with your doctor before taking a dietary supplement.

What about Herbal Supplements?

Herbal supplements are dietary supplements that come from plants. A few that you may have heard of are gingko biloba, ginseng, echinacea, and black cohosh. Researchers are looking at using herbal supplements to prevent or treat some health problems. It's too soon to know if herbal supplements are both safe and useful. But, studies of some have not shown benefits.

Are Dietary Supplements Safe?

Scientists are still working to answer this question. The U.S. Food and Drug Administration (FDA) checks prescription medicines, such as antibiotics or blood pressure medicines, to make sure they are safe and do what they promise. The same is true for over-the-counter drugs like pain and cold medicines.

But the FDA does not consider dietary supplements to be medicines. The FDA does not watch over dietary supplements in the same way it does prescription medicines. The Federal Government does not regularly test what is in dietary supplements. So, just because you see a dietary supplement on a store shelf does not mean it is safe or that it even does what the label says it will or contains what the label says it contains.

If the FDA receives reports of possible problems with a supplement, it will issue warnings about products that are clearly unsafe. The FDA may also take these supplements off the market. The Federal Trade Commission looks into reports of ads that might misrepresent what dietary supplements do.

A few private groups, such as the U.S. Pharmacopeia (USP), NSF International, ConsumerLab.com, and the Natural Products Association (NPA), have their own "seals of approval" for dietary supplements. To get such a seal, products must be made by following good manufacturing procedures, must contain what is listed on the label, and must not have harmful levels of things that don't belong there, like lead.

What's Best for Me?

If you are thinking about using dietary supplements:

- **Learn.** Find out as much as you can about any dietary supplement you might take. Talk to your doctor, your pharmacist, or a registered dietitian. A supplement that seemed to help your neighbor might not work for you. If you are reading fact sheets or checking websites, be aware of the source of the information. Could the writer or group profit from the sale of a particular supplement? For more information from the National Institute on Aging about choosing reliable health information websites, see *For More Information.*

- **Remember.** Just because something is said to be "natural" doesn't also mean it is either safe or good for you. It could have side effects. It might make a medicine your doctor prescribed for you either weaker or stronger.

- **Tell your doctor.** He or she needs to know if you decide to go ahead and use a dietary supplement. Do not diagnose or treat your health condition without first checking with your doctor.

- **Buy wisely.** Choose brands that your doctor, dietitian, or pharmacist says are trustworthy. Don't buy dietary supplements with ingredients you don't need. Don't assume that more of something that might be good for you is even better for you.

- **Check the science.** Make sure any claim made about a dietary supplement is based on scientific proof. The company making the dietary supplement should be able to send you information on the safety and/or effectiveness of the ingredients in a product, which you can then discuss with your doctor. Remember that if something sounds too good to be true, it probably is.

What Can I Do to Stay Healthy?

Here's what one active older person does:

When she turned 60, Pearl decided she wanted to stay healthy and active as long as possible. She was careful about what she ate. She became more physically active. Now she takes a long, brisk walk 3 or 4 times a week. In bad weather, she joins the mall walkers at the local shopping mall. When it's nice outside, Pearl works in her garden. When she was younger, Pearl stopped smoking and started using a seatbelt. She's even learning how to use a computer to find healthy recipes. Last month, she danced at her granddaughter's wedding. Pearl is 84 years old.

Try following Pearl's example—stick to a healthy diet, be physically active, keep your mind active, don't smoke, see your doctor regularly, and, in most cases, only use dietary supplements suggested by your doctor or pharmacist.

For More Information

Here are some helpful resources:

Department of Agriculture
Food and Nutrition Information Center
National Agricultural Library
10301 Baltimore Avenue, Room 105
Beltsville, MD 20705-2351
301-504-5414
www.nal.usda.gov/fnic

Federal Trade Commission
600 Pennsylvania Avenue, NW
Washington, DC 20580
877-382-4357 (toll-free)
202-326-2222
www.ftc.gov/healthclaims

Food and Drug Administration
Center for Food Safety and
Applied Nutrition
5100 Paint Branch Parkway HFS-555

College Park, MD 20740-3835
888-723-3366 (toll-free)
www.cfsan.fda.gov
National Center for Complementary and Alternative Medicine
NCCAM Clearinghouse
Box 7923
Gaithersburg, MD 20898
888-644-6226 (toll-free)
866-464-3615 (TTY/toll-free)
www.nccam.nih.gov

National Library of Medicine MedlinePlus
www.medlineplus.gov

Office of Dietary Supplements
6100 Executive Boulevard
Room 3B01, MSC 7517
Bethesda, MD 20892-7517
301-435-2920
www.ods.od.nih.gov

The Federal Government has several other websites with information on nutrition, including:

www.nutrition.gov—learn more about healthy eating, food shopping, assistance programs, and nutritionrelated health subjects.

www.mypyramid.gov—information about the *Dietary Guidelines for Americans*.

For information on exercise, nutrition, and health quackery and other resources on health and aging, contact:

National Institute on Aging Information Center
P.O. Box 8057
Gaithersburg, MD 20898-8057
800-222-2225 (toll-free)
800-222-4225 (TTY/toll-free)
www.nia.nih.gov

www.nia.nih.gov/Espanol

To sign up for regular email alerts about new publications and other information from the NIA, go to *www.nia.nih.gov/HealthInformation.*

Visit NIHSeniorHealth (*www.nihseniorhealth.gov*), a senior-friendly website from the National Institute on Aging and National Library of Medicine. This website has health information for older adults. Special features make it simple to use. For example, you can click on a button to have the text read out loud or to make the type larger.

In: Dietary Supplements: Primer and FDA...   ISBN: 978-1-60741-891-7
Editors: Timothy H. Riley   © 2010 Nova Science Publishers, Inc.

Chapter 2

DIETARY SUPPLEMENTS: FDA SHOULD TAKE FURTHER ACTIONS TO IMPROVE OVERSIGHT AND CONSUMER UNDERSTANDING

Government Accountability Office

WHY GAO DID THIS STUDY

Dietary supplements and foods with added dietary ingredients, such as vitamins and herbs, constitute multibillion dollar industries. Past reports on the Food and Drug Administration's (FDA) regulation of these products raised concerns about product safety and the availability of reliable information. Since then, FDA published draft guidance on requirements for reporting adverse events—which are harmful effects or illnesses—and Current Good Manufacturing Practice regulations for dietary supplements. GAO was asked to examine FDA's (1) actions to respond to the new serious adverse event reporting requirements, (2) ability to identify and act on concerns about the safety of dietary supplements, (3) ability to identify and act on concerns about the safety of foods with added dietary ingredients, and (4) actions to ensure that consumers have useful information about the safety and efficacy of supplements.

What GAO Recommends

GAO recommends that the Secretary of Health and Human Services direct the Commissioner of the FDA to request additional authority to oversee dietary supplements, issue guidance on new dietary ingredients and to clarify the boundary between dietary supplements and foods with added dietary ingredients, and take steps to improve consumer understanding of dietary supplements. In commenting on this report, FDA generally agreed with GAO's recommendations.

To view the full product, including the scope and methodology, click on GAO-09-250. For more information, contact Lisa Shames at (202) 512-3841 or shamesl@gao.gov.

What GAO Found

FDA has made several changes in response to the new serious adverse event reporting requirements and has subsequently received an increased number of reports. For example, FDA has modified its data system, issued draft guidance, and conducted outreach to industry. Since mandatory reporting went into effect on December 22, 2007, FDA has seen a threefold increase in the number of all adverse event reports received by the agency compared with the previous year. For example, from January through October 2008, FDA received 948 adverse event reports—596 of which were mandatory reports submitted by industry—compared with 298 received over the same time period in 2007. Although FDA has received a greater number of reports since the requirements went into effect, underreporting remains a concern, and the agency has further actions planned to facilitate adverse event reporting.

FDA has taken some steps to identify and act upon safety concerns related to dietary supplements; however, several factors limit the agency's ability to detect concerns and remove products from the market. For example, FDA has limited information on the number and location of dietary supplement firms, the types of products currently available in the marketplace, and information about moderate and mild adverse events reported to industry. Additionally, FDA dedicates relatively few resources to oversight activities, such as providing guidance to industry regarding notification requirements for products containing new dietary ingredients. Also, once FDA has identified a safety concern, the agency's ability to remove a product from the market is hindered by a lack of mandatory recall authority and the difficult process of demonstrating significant or unreasonable risk for specific ingredients.

Although FDA has taken some actions when foods contain unsafe dietary ingredients, certain factors may allow potentially unsafe products to reach consumers. FDA may not know when a company has made an unsupported or incorrect determination about whether an added dietary ingredient in a product is generally recognized as safe until after the product becomes available to consumers because companies are not required to notify FDA of their self-determinations. In addition, the boundary between dietary supplements and conventional foods containing dietary ingredients is not always clear, and some food products could be marketed as dietary supplements to circumvent the safety standard required for food additives.

FDA has taken limited steps to educate consumers about dietary supplements, and studies and experts indicate that consumer understanding is lacking. While FDA has conducted some outreach, these initiatives have reached a relatively small proportion of dietary supplement consumers. Additionally, surveys and experts indicate that consumers are not well-informed about the safety and efficacy of dietary supplements and have difficulty interpreting labels on these products. Without a clear understanding of the safety, efficacy, and labeling of dietary supplements, consumers may be exposed to greater health risks associated with the uninformed use of these products.

January 29, 2009
The Honorable Henry A. Waxman
Chairman
The Honorable John D. Dingell
Chairman Emeritus
Committee on Energy and Commerce
House of Representatives

The Honorable Bart Stupak
Chairman
Subcommittee on Oversight and Investigations
Committee on Energy and Commerce
House of Representatives

The Honorable Richard J.
Durbin United States Senate

Dietary supplements and foods containing added dietary ingredients, such as vitamins and herbs, constitute growing multibillion dollar industries. Sales of dietary supplements alone reached approximately $23.7 billion in 2007, and data from the 2007 National Health Interview Survey show that over half of all U.S. adults consume dietary supplements. In 1994, there were approximately 4,000 dietary supplement products on the market, whereas an industry source estimated that, in 2008, about 75,000 dietary supplement products were available to consumers. Similarly, food products—such as fortified cereals and energy drinks—that contain added dietary ingredients are in the marketplace in unprecedented numbers, and consumers are expected to spend increasing amounts on these products over the next several years.

The Food and Drug Administration (FDA) regulates dietary supplements under provisions of the Federal Food, Drug, and Cosmetic Act, as amended by the Dietary Supplement Health and Education Act of 1994 (DSHEA). DSHEA defines dietary supplements as products that, among other things, are intended for ingestion to supplement the diet, labeled as a dietary supplement, and not represented as a conventional food or as a sole item of a meal or diet. They must also contain one or more dietary ingredients. DSHEA does not require manufacturers to register with FDA or identify the products they manufacture or the ingredients of those products. However, all food facilities, including manufacturers and distributors of dietary supplements, were required to register with FDA no later than December 12, 2003, under the Public Health Security and Bioterrorism Preparedness and Response Act of 2002 and implementing regulations. This includes an initial registration with FDA and updates within 60 days of any changes in information. Registration must include the name and address of the facility and an emergency contact, and facilities that manufacture or sell certain types of products, such as vitamins, must self-identify as such.

Under DSHEA, dietary supplements are broadly presumed safe, and FDA does not have the authority to require them to be approved for safety and efficacy before they enter the market, as it does for drugs. However, a dietary supplement manufacturer or distributor of a supplement with a "new dietary ingredient"—an ingredient that was not marketed in the United States before October 15, 1994—may be required to notify FDA at least 75 days before marketing the product, depending on the history of use of the ingredient. For the most part, FDA relies on post-market surveillance efforts—such as monitoring adverse event reports it receives from companies, health care practitioners, and individuals; reviewing consumer complaints; and conducting facility inspections—to identify potential safety concerns related to dietary supplements. Once a safety concern is identified, FDA must demonstrate that the dietary supplement presents a significant or unreasonable risk, or is otherwise adulterated, before it can be removed from the market. According to several experts we spoke with, this regulatory approach has fallen short in protecting U.S. consumers in the past. For example, while FDA was successful, in 2004, in banning ephedrine alkaloids (ephedra)—a dietary ingredient used for weight loss and bodybuilding, among other things—the ban became effective only after FDA had received thousands of reports of adverse events, including a number of deaths, and 10 years after the agency issued its first advisory.

Since ephedra was banned, several changes have occurred in the regulation of dietary supplements. For example, the Federal Food, Drug, and Cosmetic Act, as amended by the Dietary Supplement and Nonprescription Drug Consumer Protection Act, requires companies that receive a serious adverse event report to submit information about the event to FDA, beginning in December 2007. As defined in the act, serious adverse events include any health-related events that result in, for example, a death, life-threatening experience, inpatient hospitalization, birth defect, or which require, based on reasonable medical judgment, a medical or surgical intervention to prevent these serious outcomes. While the act does not require companies to report moderate or mild adverse events, such as gastrointestinal distress or headaches, companies may do so voluntarily. In addition, health care practitioners and consumers can submit voluntary reports of serious, moderate, and mild adverse events. Additionally, in an effort to improve the consistency and safety of dietary supplements, in June 2007, FDA established its Current Good Manufacturing Practice regulations describing the conditions under which supplements must be manufactured, packed, and held. These requirements are being implemented in phases, based on company size, and will be fully in effect by 2010.

In addition to regulating the safety and labeling of dietary supplements, FDA also conducts outreach to consumers about these products. While the Federal Food, Drug, and Cosmetic Act does not explicitly require FDA to conduct consumer education, according to the agency, it has some responsibility for doing so.

FDA also regulates foods with added dietary ingredients under provisions set out in the Federal Food, Drug, and Cosmetic Act. The act generally requires that when a company adds an ingredient to a food product, that ingredient must either be generally recognized as safe (GRAS) or go through FDA's review and approval process as a food additive. With some exceptions, the company is responsible for determining that the ingredient meets the GRAS standard or, failing this, for having it approved as a food additive. The GRAS standard is defined as a general recognition among qualified experts that the substance is reasonably certain to not be harmful under its intended conditions of use; such recognition can come through scientific procedures, or for substances in use prior to 1958, through experience based on common use in food. If the added ingredient is GRAS, the company may add the ingredient to a food product without notifying FDA, although some do so voluntarily. In most instances, if the ingredient does not meet the GRAS standard, the company must petition FDA for approval of the ingredient as a food additive, which also requires companies to demonstrate a reasonable certainty that the ingredient is not harmful under the intended conditions of use. According to FDA, meeting the safety standard for a food additive requires the same quantity and quality of scientific evidence as is needed to satisfy the GRAS standard.

In July 2000, we reported concerns about the safety of dietary supplements and foods with added dietary ingredients, as well as about the accuracy of health-related claims on product labels and in advertising.[1] More specifically, we reported that consumers faced health risks because federal laws and agencies' efforts did not effectively and consistently ensure that products were safe. Furthermore, we found that consumers did not consistently receive clear, scientifically supported information concerning products' health benefits so they could make informed dietary choices. To help ensure that dietary supplements and related products are safe and that consumers receive accurate information about the products, we made six recommendations to FDA. FDA has implemented two of these recommendations but has not fully implemented the remaining four, which deal largely with providing regulations or other information clarifying industry responsibilities.

At your request, this report examines FDA's (1) actions to respond to the new serious adverse event reporting requirements; (2) ability to identify and act on concerns about the safety of dietary supplements; (3) ability to identify and act on concerns about the safety of foods with added dietary ingredients; and (4) actions to educate consumers about the safety, efficacy, and labeling of dietary supplements.

For this report, dietary supplement means a product intended for human consumption and does not include products for veterinary use. Additionally, for this report, dietary ingredient means an ingredient that is included in the dietary supplement definition in DSHEA, such as vitamins, minerals, and herbs or other botanicals. To identify FDA's actions to respond to the new serious adverse event reporting requirements, we reviewed FDA's guidance on reporting requirements for industry and internal procedures for compiling and tracking adverse event reports; analyzed the number of reports received before and after the requirements went into effect; and reviewed plans for improving adverse event reporting. To examine

FDA's ability to identify and act on safety concerns associated with dietary supplements, we assessed FDA's laws and regulations; analyzed data on FDA's oversight actions, such as inspections, import screenings and enforcement activities; and reviewed FDA resources dedicated to dietary supplements. To examine FDA's ability to identify and act on concerns about the safety of foods with added dietary ingredients, we reviewed laws and regulations regarding food additives, as well as FDA's procedures for identifying and acting on concerns about the safety of foods with added dietary ingredients. To determine what FDA has done to educate consumers about the safety, efficacy, and labeling of dietary supplements, we reviewed FDA's consumer outreach initiatives and analyzed FDA's and others' data on consumer understanding of dietary supplements. In addition, to address all of our objectives, we interviewed a wide range of stakeholders, including officials from federal and state agencies, industry and trade organizations, consumer advocacy groups, academia, poison control centers, and foreign governments. To assess the reliability of the data from FDA's databases used in this report, we reviewed related documentation, examined the data to identify obvious errors or inconsistencies, and worked with agency officials to identify any data problems. We determined the data to be sufficiently reliable for the purposes of this report. A more detailed description of our objectives, scope, and methodology is presented in appendix I.

We conducted this performance audit from December 2007 to January 2009, in accordance with generally accepted government auditing standards. Those standards require that we plan and perform the audit to obtain sufficient, appropriate evidence to provide a reasonable basis for our findings and conclusions based on our audit objectives. We believe that the evidence obtained provides a reasonable basis for our findings and conclusions based on our audit objectives.

RESULTS IN BRIEF

In 2007, FDA took several actions in response to the new serious adverse event reporting requirements for dietary supplements and has subsequently received an increased number of reports. Specifically, FDA has incorporated the mandatory reports into its existing data system for compiling, tracking, and reviewing adverse event reports. FDA has also issued draft guidance and conducted outreach to industry regarding the new reporting requirements. For example, in October 2007, FDA provided companies with a form and instructions for submitting mandatory serious adverse event reports and issued draft guidance outlining requirements and recommendations for reporting, recordkeeping, and records access. Furthermore, FDA has worked with industry associations to increase awareness of the new reporting requirements. Since mandatory reporting requirements went into effect, the agency has seen a threefold increase in the number of all adverse events reported compared with the previous year. For example, from January through October 2008, FDA received 948 adverse event reports, compared with 298 received over the same time period in 2007. Of the 948 adverse event reports, 596 were mandatory reports of serious adverse events submitted by industry; the remaining 352 were voluntary reports, which include all moderate and mild adverse events reported and any serious adverse events reported by health care practitioners and consumers directly to FDA. However, FDA recently estimated that the actual number of total adverse events—including mild, moderate, and serious—related to dietary supplements per year is over 50,000, which suggests that underreporting of adverse events limits the amount of information FDA receives. To facilitate adverse event reporting for all FDA-regulated products, FDA is currently developing MedWatchPlus, an interactive Web-based portal intended to simplify the reporting process and reduce the time and cost associated with reviewing paper reports.

Although FDA has used varied approaches—such as analyzing adverse events and conducting inspections—to identify safety concerns and has taken some actions—such as detaining certain potentially unsafe imported products—in response to these concerns, several factors limit FDA's ability to further identify and act on safety concerns. First, FDA's ability to identify safety concerns is hindered by a lack of information. For example, while all dietary supplement companies must register with FDA as food facilities to provide their name and address, some companies—such as those specializing exclusively in herbal products—are not required to identify themselves as dietary supplement companies. In addition, companies are not required to provide FDA with information on the products they sell, such as the product name and ingredients. As a result, FDA has limited information on the companies and products it is required to regulate, and more complete information could help FDA analyze adverse event reports. Moreover, dietary supplement companies are required to report only serious adverse events. FDA officials have noted that receiving adverse event reports for moderate and mild events could improve the agency's ability to assess safety-related signals from adverse event data. Second, in comparison to other regulated products, FDA dedicates relatively few resources to dietary supplement oversight activities. For example, FDA has conducted relatively few dietary supplement inspections and has not developed guidance for industry regarding key safety-related aspects of DSHEA in a timely manner. In particular, FDA has not yet issued guidance to clarify new dietary ingredient notification requirements. Third, once FDA has identified a safety concern, its ability to efficiently and effectively remove a product from the market is limited. For example, FDA lacks mandatory recall authority, and FDA's ability to ban an unsafe ingredient has proven difficult because the Federal Food, Drug, and Cosmetic Act requires that the agency demonstrate a significant or unreasonable risk or that the dietary supplement is otherwise adulterated. This statutory requirement is exacerbated by limited scientific research and underreporting of adverse events. Although FDA has taken some steps, such as drafting guidance for industry on reporting serious adverse events and establishing its Current Good Manufacturing Practice regulations, to improve the oversight of dietary supplements over the past several years, consumers remain vulnerable to risks posed by potentially unsafe products.

Similar to dietary supplements, while FDA has taken some actions, such as issuing warnings, when foods contain unsafe dietary ingredients, certain factors may allow some unsafe products to reach consumers. For example, FDA may not know when a company has made an unsupported or incorrect GRAS determination about an added dietary ingredient in a product until after the product becomes available to consumers because companies are not required to notify FDA of their self-determinations. In addition, the boundary between dietary supplements and foods with added dietary ingredients is not always clear, and some food products could be marketed as dietary supplements to circumvent the safety standard required for food additives. For example, in August 2007, FDA identified a company marketing an iced tea mix containing stevia—an herb that has not been approved as a food additive because of potential safety concerns, including reproductive and cardiovascular effects. FDA issued a warning to the company, and the company changed the product label to classify the product as a dietary supplement rather than a food so that it could continue to add stevia to its product. As a dietary supplement, FDA does not have the authority to require that the safety of the product be approved. Finally, FDA conducts limited monitoring of foods with added dietary ingredients. According to FDA, it does not track these products separately from other conventional foods, and the current regulatory framework is sufficient to identify and act on safety concerns related to these products. Some stakeholders we spoke with noted that safety risks associated with foods containing added dietary ingredients that meet the GRAS standard or have been approved as food additives are generally low. However, some stakeholders expressed concerns about certain products, such as energy drinks, and adding botanicals to foods.

FDA has taken limited steps to educate consumers about the safety, efficacy, and labeling of dietary supplements, and studies and experts indicate that consumer understanding about these products is lacking. While FDA has conducted some consumer outreach, such as distributing brochures and providing information its Web site, these initiatives have reached a relatively small proportion of consumers using dietary supplements. For instance, a 2004 brochure developed in conjunction with the National Institutes of Health (NIH) had a distribution of 40,000 paper copies and received approximately 171,000 page views on the Web. However, data from the 2007 National Health Interview Survey show that over half of U.S. adults—or at least 114 million individuals— take dietary supplements. While officials noted that the agency must continually market its desired messages to effectively educate consumers, FDA's Center for Food Safety and Applied Nutrition (CFSAN) currently is not planning any new consumer education initiatives for dietary supplements. In addition, agency officials stated that FDA does not evaluate the effectiveness of its outreach efforts; however, surveys and experts indicate that consumers are not well-informed about factors that can affect the safety and efficacy of dietary supplements. For example, a 2002 Harris Poll indicated that a majority of adults believe that a government agency approves dietary supplements before products are marketed to consumers. Studies also suggest that the labeling of dietary supplements can be confusing to consumers. For example, in 2003, the Department of Health and Human Services' Inspector General reported that dietary supplement labels often do not present information in a manner that facilitates consumer understanding.[2] Without a clear understanding of the safety, efficacy, and labeling of dietary supplements, consumers are exposed to risks— such as potentially harmful drug-supplement interactions—associated with the uninformed use of these products.

To improve the information available to FDA for identifying safety concerns, we are recommending that the Secretary of the Department of Health and Human Services direct the Commissioner of FDA to seek additional authority to require dietary supplement facilities to self-identify as part of existing registration requirements, provide a list of their products and a copy of the labels, and report all adverse events related to dietary supplements. To better enable FDA to regulate dietary supplements with new dietary ingredients, we are recommending that the Secretary of the Department of Health and Human Services direct the Commissioner of FDA to issue guidance to clarify when an ingredient is considered a new dietary ingredient, what evidence is needed to document the safety of new dietary ingredients, and appropriate methods for establishing ingredient identity. To help ensure that companies follow the appropriate laws and regulations, we are recommending that the Secretary of the Department of Health and Human Services direct the Commissioner of FDA to provide guidance to industry to clarify when products should be marketed as either dietary supplements or conventional foods formulated with added dietary ingredients. We made a similar recommendation in our July 2000 report, but, according to FDA, it did not implement the recommendation because of resource constraints and competing agency priorities and activities. To improve consumer understanding about dietary supplements and better leverage existing resources, we are recommending that the Secretary of the Department of Health and Human Services direct the Commissioner of FDA to coordinate with stakeholder groups to identify additional mechanisms to educate consumers, implement these mechanisms, and assess their effectiveness. In commenting on our draft report, FDA generally agreed with our recommendations.

BACKGROUND

According to the *Nutrition Business Journal*, the dietary supplement industry is growing, and total sales were about $23.7 billion in 2007, as shown in figure 1. Top selling supplements in 2007 included multivitamins, sports nutrition powders and formulas, and calcium, according to the *Nutrition Business Journal*. In addition, one of the areas of greatest growth in supplements within the United States in 2007 was among weight loss products. Projections through 2011 show that growth in the industry is expected to continue, in large part because of the aging population and an increasing interest in personal health and wellness.

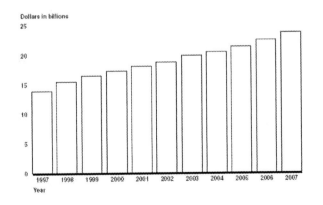

Figure 1. Total Sales of Dietary Supplements in the United States from 1997 through 2007

Source: GAO *analysis of Nutrition Business Journal data.*

Over time, several key events have shaped the regulation of dietary supplements, as shown in table 1. Significantly, Congress passed DSHEA, which amended the Federal Food, Drug, and Cosmetic Act and created a new regulatory category, safety standard, and other requirements for supplements. Under DSHEA, dietary supplements are generally presumed safe. With the exception of the banned dietary ingredient, ephedra, companies may sell otherwise lawful products containing any dietary ingredient that was marketed in the United States prior to October 15, 1994—referred to as "grandfathered ingredients"—without notifying FDA. Ingredients that were not marketed before this date are considered new dietary ingredients. A dietary supplement containing a new dietary ingredient must meet one of the two following requirements: (1) it contains only dietary ingredients that have been "present in the food supply as an article used for food in a form in which the food has not been chemically altered" or (2) there is evidence that the dietary ingredient is reasonably expected to be safe under the conditions of use recommended or suggested in the product's labeling. In addition, companies planning to market a dietary supplement with a new dietary ingredient that only meets the second requirement must notify FDA of the evidence that is the basis of the determination at least 75 days before marketing the supplement.

Table 1. Key Events in the Regulation of Dietary Supplements

Year	Key event
1990	The Nutrition Labeling and Education Act of 1990 amended the Federal Food, Drug, and Cosmetic Act to require most foods, including dietary supplements, to bear nutrition labeling.
1994	DSHEA amended the Federal Food, Drug, and Cosmetic Act to create a new regulatory category, safety standard, labeling requirements, and other rules for dietary supplements. Under DSHEA, dietary supplements are generally presumed to be safe.
2002	The Public Health Security and Bioterrorism Preparedness and Response Act of 2002 amended the Federal Food, Drug, and Cosmetic Act to require all food companies, including dietary supplement companies, to register with FDA no later than December 12, 2003, to provide information on the name and address of the facility and, to some extent, the types of products they manufacture or sell.
2004	FDA was successful in banning ephedra after thousands of adverse events, including a number of deaths, and a lengthy legal process.
2006	The Dietary Supplement and Nonprescription Drug Consumer Protection Act amended the Federal Food, Drug, and Cosmetic Act to require dietary supplement companies that receive a serious adverse event

	report to submit information about the event to FDA.
2007	FDA finalized its Current Good Manufacturing Practice regulations to establish quality control standards for dietary supplements. The final rule became effective on August 24, 2007, but companies have 10, 22, or 34 months from the effective date of the rule to comply, depending on company size.
2007	Serious adverse event reporting requirements for dietary supplement companies became effective on December 22.

Source: GAO.

As of December 22, 2007, dietary supplement companies are required to submit any report received about a serious adverse event to FDA, as mandated by the Dietary Supplement and Nonprescription Drug Consumer Protection Act. In addition, companies can voluntarily submit reports about moderate and mild adverse events. Others, such as consumers and health care practitioners, can submit reports of serious, moderate, and mild adverse events on a voluntary basis to FDA. Prior to implementing the mandatory reporting requirements, FDA's Center for Food Safety and Applied Nutrition—which, in part, is responsible for promoting and protecting the public's health by ensuring that the nation's food supply is safe, sanitary, wholesome, and honestly labeled—had a system in place to receive voluntary reports of adverse events involving dietary supplements from all parties.

As stated in the Federal Food, Drug, and Cosmetic Act, FDA is also responsible for protecting the public health by ensuring that the labels of dietary supplements are not false or misleading. As noted in table 1, the Nutrition Labeling and Education Act of 1990 amended the Federal Food, Drug, and Cosmetic Act to require that most foods, including dietary supplements, bear nutrition labeling. In addition, DSHEA amended the Federal Food, Drug, and Cosmetic Act to add specific labeling requirements for dietary supplements and provided for optional labeling statements. Federal regulations require the following information on the labels of dietary supplements: (1) product identity (name of the dietary supplement), (2) net quantity of contents statement (amount of the dietary supplement in the package), (3) nutrition labeling, (4) ingredient list (when appropriate), and (5) name and place of business of the manufacturer, packer, or distributor. In addition, DSHEA specifies that supplements with labeling that makes disease or health-related claims must contain a disclaimer that FDA has not evaluated the claim and the product is not intended to diagnose, treat, cure, or prevent any disease.

Similar to dietary supplements, the market for foods with added dietary ingredients has been growing, and this trend is expected to continue. Foods with added dietary ingredients vary greatly, including such products as orange juice with added calcium, pasta with Omega 3, and sunflower seeds with guarana. Terms such as "functional foods" and "nutraceuticals" are sometimes used to describe foods with added dietary ingredients. However, there are no regulatory definitions for these terms, and some of these terms include foods with naturally beneficial properties beyond nutrition, such as pomegranate juice.

FDA HAS MADE CHANGES IN RESPONSE TO THE NEW SERIOUS ADVERSE EVENT REPORTING REQUIREMENTS AND HAS RECEIVED AN INCREASED NUMBER OF REPORTS

FDA has made several changes in response to the new serious adverse event reporting requirements established by law in 2006 and has subsequently received an increased number of reports. FDA has modified its existing data system and internal procedures for compiling, tracking, and reviewing adverse event reports to incorporate mandatory reporting by industry. Additionally, FDA has issued draft guidance and conducted outreach to industry regarding the new requirements. Since mandatory reporting went into effect on December 22, 2007, FDA has seen a threefold increase in the number of all adverse event reports received by the agency compared with the previous year. Although FDA received more reports overall since the reporting requirements went into effect, underreporting of adverse events remains a concern, and the agency has further actions planned to facilitate adverse event reporting by consumers, health care practitioners, and industry.

FDA Has Taken Several Actions in Response to the New Serious Adverse Event Reporting Requirements

In 2007, FDA took several actions in response to the new serious adverse event reporting requirements for dietary supplements. Specifically, FDA modified its existing database for compiling, tracking, and reviewing adverse event reports—the CFSAN Adverse Event Reporting System (CAERS)—to include data fields and instructions specifically for compiling and tracking mandatory reports. In addition, CFSAN established procedures for reviewing mandatory serious adverse event reports to determine if they meet the minimum data requirements for mandatory reports outlined in guidance to the industry.

FDA has also issued draft guidance and conducted outreach to industry regarding the new reporting requirements. In October 2007, FDA provided companies with a form and instructions for submitting mandatory serious adverse event reports and issued draft guidance describing statutory requirements and agency recommendations for reporting, recordkeeping, and records access. Additionally, in December 2007, FDA issued draft guidance on labeling requirements.

Statutory requirements outlined in draft guidance include the following:

- The manufacturer, packer, or distributor whose name appears on the dietary supplement label (responsible party) must report all serious adverse events to FDA, as well as follow up medical information received within 1 year after the initial report, within 15 business days of receipt.
- Mandatory serious adverse event reports must be submitted to FDA using the MedWatch 3500A form and should contain the following minimum data elements: an identifiable injured person, name of the person who first notified the responsible party, identity and contact information for the responsible party, a suspect dietary supplement, and a serious adverse event or fatal outcome.
- The responsible party must include a copy of the dietary supplement label related to the serious adverse event.
- The responsible party must maintain records of all adverse events reported for 6 years and must provide FDA officials with access to the records upon request during an inspection.
- Labels for dietary supplements marketed in the United States must provide a complete domestic mailing address or phone number where the responsible party may receive adverse event reports.

In addition to these requirements, FDA recommended that firms include an introductory statement on dietary supplement labels to inform consumers that the contact information provided may be used to report a serious adverse event. According to comments submitted to FDA by the three major dietary supplement industry associations, although the industry broadly supports the new mandatory reporting requirements, it disagrees with the recommended labeling changes. These industry associations cite the following three key reasons for their opposition to FDA's recommendation: (1) in their view, the changes are unnecessary and beyond Congress' intent; (2) the introductory statement may draw undue attention to the possibility of an adverse event and confuse consumers; and (3) redesigning and replacing product labels is a substantial added expense for dietary supplement companies and should have been proposed through a formal rulemaking process rather than guidance. According to an FDA official, the draft guidance regarding reporting, recordkeeping, and records access requirements is close to being finalized. In December 2008, FDA issued a revision of the draft guidance regarding labeling changes. According to FDA, before this guidance is finalized, it will need to be reviewed by the Office of Management and Budget because of its potential economic impact on industry.

FDA has also worked with industry associations to increase awareness of the new reporting requirements. For instance, FDA officials have spoken at industry-sponsored conferences and seminars to increase awareness and answer questions about the new reporting requirements. Representatives from two of the leading industry associations we spoke with stated that they were generally satisfied with FDA's outreach efforts regarding mandatory reporting.

FDA Has Received an Increased Number of Adverse Event Reports Since Mandatory Reporting Went into Effect

Since mandatory reporting requirements went into effect, the agency has seen a threefold increase in the number of all adverse events reported compared with the previous year. For example, from January through October 2008, FDA received 948 adverse event reports, compared with 298 received over the same time period in 2007. Of the 948 adverse event reports, 596 were mandatory reports of serious adverse events submitted by industry; the remaining 352 were voluntary reports, which include all moderate and mild adverse events reported and any serious adverse events reported by health care practitioners and consumers directly to FDA. As shown in figure 2, FDA received more serious adverse event reports between January 1, 2008, and October 31, 2008, than previous years, including 2003 and 2004, when FDA was receiving adverse event reports related to ephedra. Adverse event reports from January 1, 2008, through October 31, 2008, include 596 serious adverse event reports submitted by industry, 163 serious adverse events reported by others on a voluntary basis, and 189 moderate and mild adverse event reports.

Since mandatory reporting went into effect, FDA had received 596 mandatory reports of adverse events, such as serious cardiac, respiratory, and gastrointestinal disorders, as of October 31, 2008. Among other results, these events involved 9 deaths, 64 life-threatening illnesses, and 234 patient hospitalizations. As shown in table 2, 66 percent of serious adverse event reports were associated with dietary supplements that either contained a combination of types of products, such as a product containing both vitamins and herbals, or could not be categorized under one of FDA's other product classifications, and 40 percent were associated with vitamins. However, according to FDA, because of variability in the quality and detail of information in reports and the lack of a control group, the agency cannot necessarily determine a causal relationship between an adverse event and the dietary supplement associated with the event. Appendix II provides further detail on adverse event reports related to dietary supplements received by FDA from January 1, 2003 through August 6, 2008.

Although FDA has received a greater number of reports since mandatory reporting requirements went into effect, FDA recently estimated that the actual number of total adverse events—including serious, moderate, and mild—related to dietary supplements per year is over 50,000.[3] This estimate suggests that underreporting of adverse events limits the amount of information that FDA receives regarding safety concerns related to dietary supplements or their ingredients and, according to FDA, this can negatively impact the agency's ability to identify safety concerns.

Experts have cited several possible reasons for underreporting related to dietary supplements, including reduced attribution of adverse effects to supplements due to the assumption that all dietary supplements are safe, the reluctance of consumers to report dietary supplement use to physicians, the failure to recognize chronic or cumulative toxic effects from their use, and a cumbersome reporting process. To facilitate adverse event reporting for any FDA-regulated products, FDA is currently developing MedWatchPlus, an interactive Web-based portal intended to simplify the reporting process and reduce the time and cost associated with reviewing paper reports. For example, according to FDA planning documents, MedWatchPlus would simplify the reporting process by providing a single Internet portal for consumers, health care providers, and industry to report an adverse event. Furthermore, the proposed interactive format will prompt reporters to provide relevant information based on the type of products involved in the adverse event—thereby facilitating reporting and improving the quality of information FDA receives. Once an event is reported, the information would be automatically routed to the relevant FDA centers based on the type of product involved. Testing and release of the interactive questionnaire phase of the project is currently expected in 2009.

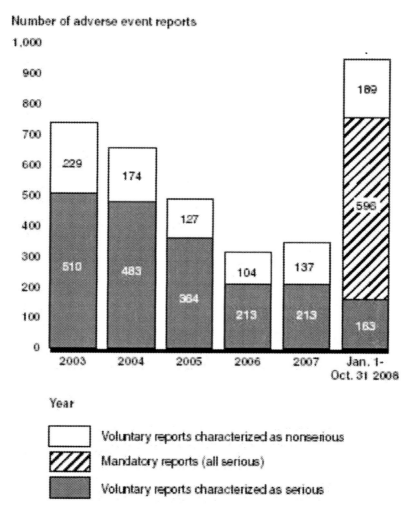

Figure 2. The Number of Dietary Supplement-Related Adverse Event Reports to CAERS from January 1, 2003, to October 31, 2008

Note: There were 36 reports that did not include information about seriousness in 2003. FDA officials noted that, prior to the ban on ephedra in 2004, the agency received a heightened number of adverse event reports due to products containing ephedra. Although mandatory reporting went into effect on December 22, 2007, FDA did not receive its first mandatory report until January 2008.

Table 2. Number of Cases with Mandatory Reported Adverse Event Outcomes by Dietary Supplement Product Classification, from December 22, 2007, through October 31, 2008

Dietary supplement product classification	Number of serious adverse events reported, from December 22, 2007, through October 31, 2008	Percentage of all serious adverse events reported
Combination products and products not elsewhere classified	391	65.6%
Vitamin	240	40.3
Mineral	111	18.6
Fats and lipid substances	55	9.2
Herbal and botanical (other than tea)	24	4.0
Fiber	20	3.4
Herbal and botanical teas	15	2.5
Protein	9	1.5
Animal by-products and extracts	1	0.2%
Total	596[a]	

Source: FDA.

[a]Total does not add because some adverse event reports involved more than one product and are counted in more than one subcategory. For example, according to FDA, if a consumer was taking both a vitamin C supplement and an echinacea supplement when the adverse event took place, the event would be classified under both "vitamin" and "herbal and botanical." If the consumer was taking a single product containing both vitamin C and echinacea, the event would be classified under "combination products."

ALTHOUGH FDA HAS TAKEN SOME STEPS TO IDENTIFY AND ACT ON CONCERNS ABOUT THE SAFETY OF DIETARY SUPPLEMENTS, SEVERAL FACTORS LIMIT ITS OVERSIGHT

FDA has taken some steps—such as analyzing adverse event reports and detaining certain potentially unsafe imported products—to identify and act upon safety concerns related to dietary supplements. However, several factors limit the agency's ability to detect concerns and efficiently and effectively remove products from the market. For example, FDA has limited information on the number and location of dietary supplement firms, the identity and ingredients of products currently available in the marketplace, and mild and moderate adverse events reported to industry. Additionally, FDA dedicates relatively few resources to dietary supplement oversight activities compared with other FDA-regulated products. Moreover, once the agency has identified a safety concern, the agency's ability to efficiently and effectively remove a product from the market is hindered by a lack of mandatory recall authority and the difficulty of establishing adulteration for dietary supplement products under the significant or unreasonable risk standard. Although FDA has taken some steps, such as drafting guidance for industry on reporting serious adverse events and establishing its Current Good Manufacturing Practice regulations, to improve the oversight of dietary supplements over the past several years, consumers remain vulnerable to risks posed by potentially unsafe products.

FDA Has Taken Some Actions to Identify and Act on Concerns about the Safety of Dietary Supplements

FDA uses a variety of approaches to identify potential safety concerns related to dietary supplements. For example, FDA may identify concerns through surveillance actions such as monitoring adverse event reports and consumer complaints, screening imports, and conducting inspections. For instance, during almost half of the 909 inspections conducted at dietary supplement firms from fiscal year 2002 through May 6, 2008, FDA and its partners at the state level identified potential problems, such as a lack of quality control and unsanitary conditions. Table 3 provides examples of FDA surveillance related to dietary supplements. For more detailed information on FDA's actions to identify potential safety concerns, see appendix II.

Table 3. Examples of FDA Surveillance to Identify Safety Concerns

Surveillance actions	
Monitoring adverse events	FDA received 3,502 adverse event reports related to dietary supplements from January 1, 2003 through October 31, 2008. The top three outcomes associated with these cases were hospitalization (32 percent), nonserious illness or injury (28 percent), and serious illness or injury (25 percent).[a]

Monitoring consumer complaints	FDA received 1,018 consumer complaints from fiscal year 2001 through July 3, 2008. Forty-two percent of these complaints involved adverse symptoms. Consumer com-plaints involving adverse symptoms triggered 236 active surveillance operations, including inspections and sample collections.
Screening imports	FDA reviewed 616,464 import entry lines of dietary supplements from fiscal year 2002 through March 24, 2008, and either sampled or examined, on average, approxima-tely 3 to 5 percent of the imported entry lines entering the country.[b]
Conducting inspections	FDA conducted 804 inspections, and state partners conducted 105 inspections, of domestic dietary supplement firms from fiscal years 2002 through 2008. Investigators identified potential problems, such as a lack of quality control and unsanitary conditions, in 49 percent of these inspections.

Source: GAO analysis of FDA data.

[a] An adverse event report case may have more than one reported outcome.

[b] According to FDA, an entry line is each portion of an import shipment that is listed as a separate item on an entry document. Items in an import entry having different tariff descriptions must be listed separately.

In addition, FDA monitors the Internet to identify products that purport to be dietary supplements but may be fraudulently promoted for treating diseases. According to FDA, such products pose a threat to public health because the disease prevention and treatment claims often persuade consumers to delay or forgo medical diagnosis and treatment. FDA officials also told us they identify safety concerns by obtaining information from other agencies at the state, federal, and international level; reviewing scientific literature; sponsoring safety-related research; and targeting safety-related investigations on particular classes of products. For instance, according to FDA, the agency used adverse event information from the Florida Department of Health to issue a consumer warning about the product "Total Body Formula." FDA officials also described current safety-related investigations it initiated targeting specific classes of products, such as ephedra substitutes; male potency enhancers that contain undeclared active pharmaceutical ingredients; and products making misleading health claims to prevent or cure serious illnesses such as diabetes, sudden acute respiratory syndrome, and influenza. For example, officials said they are currently contracting with the University of California at Los Angeles to monitor adverse event reporting related to ephedra substitutes. In addition, FDA is conducting animal testing through the National Center for Toxicological Research to examine interactions among weight loss supplement ingredients, according to agency officials.

Once FDA has identified a potential safety concern, the agency has several options available for taking action. According to FDA officials, products or ingredients of greatest concern for public health generally will be subject to either administrative or judicial enforcement actions, whereas FDA will take advisory actions against products of lower public health risk. FDA officials also noted that, if a firm does not correct violations in response to an advisory action, FDA may pursue an enforcement action against the firm. Table 4 provides examples of FDA administrative and enforcement actions related to dietary supplements. For more detailed information on FDA's actions in response to identified safety concerns, see appendix II.

In addition to taking enforcement action on its own, FDA may pursue enforcement action in conjunction with another federal agency, such as the Federal Trade Commission, which has enforcement responsibility with regard to dietary supplement advertising. For example, as part of the FDA's Consumer Health Information for Better Nutrition initiative launched in 2002, FDA and the Federal Trade Commission took joint enforcement actions against several marketers of dietary supplement products making unsubstantiated treatment claims for diseases such as emphysema, diabetes, Alzheimer's disease, cancer, and multiple sclerosis. In addition, industry has also initiated some measures to address unsubstantiated claims. For example, based on monitoring efforts and company referrals, the National Advertising Division of the Council of Better Business Bureaus reviews advertising claims for accuracy and then recommends changes to companies as necessary. This program is currently funded through a series of multiyear grants from the Council for Responsible Nutrition.

Table 4. Examples of FDA Actions in Response to Identified Safety Concerns

Advisory actions	
Hold regulatory meeting with the firm	FDA officials may meet with firm representatives to discuss concerns and request voluntary action; however, FDA does not collect agencywide data on these meetings.
Issue firm a warning	FDA issued 293 warning letters citing 534 violations regarding dietary supplements from fiscal years 2002 through 2007. Seventy percent of these violations related to dietary supplements that FDA determined were either unapproved new drugs or misbranded drugs.
Issue consumer alerts	FDA had posted 12 consumer alerts on its Web site since 1999, including warnings for kava, aristolochic acid, and St. John's wort, among others, as of November 21, 2008.

Issue advisory to industry	FDA had posted letters to industry advising against the marketing of products containing aristolochic acid, comfrey, androstenedione, Lipokinetix, and ephedra, as of November 21, 2008.
Administrative and judicial enforcement actions to remove a product from the market	
Work with company on a voluntary product recall	At least 45 recalls related to dangerous or defective dietary supplement products that posed a serious health concern were initiated from fiscal years 2003 through 2008. Of these recalls, 27 were due to the unapproved presence of pharmaceutical ingredients in the supplement products.
Detain/refuse the product if imported	FDA detained 3,225 dietary supplement import entry lines from fiscal year 2002 through March 24, 2008. Fifty percent of the detentions were due to the potential presence of a poisonous or unsafe substance. Over this same period, FDA refused 3,604 lines of dietary supplements, citing 5,560 violations. Twenty-five percent of the violations were due to the potential presence of an unsafe substance.
Pursue legal action against the firm	FDA initiated action for 27 seizures and 6 injunctions from fiscal year 2002 through July 18, 2008. Nineteen of the seizures and 6 of the injunctions regarded products promoted to treat, cure, or prevent diseases. FDA had filed criminal charges or won convictions in 19 cases since fiscal year 2002, as of July 31, 2008.
Ban ingredient	FDA banned one ingredient—ephedra—in 2004, almost 10 years after issuing its first advisory. FDA has not banned any other dietary supplement ingredients.

Source: GAO analysis of FDA data.

FDA officials also noted that the agency plans to expand dietary supplement oversight in the near term. In particular, FDA will add dietary supplement inspections as an option for its formal state contract agreements in 2009, which should increase the number of dietary supplement inspections performed by state officials on FDA's behalf, according to FDA officials.[4] To further increase the number of inspections, FDA is also exploring third-party certification as part of its *Food Protection Plan: An Integrated Strategy for Protecting the Nation's Food Supply*.[5] To improve the agency's Internet surveillance, FDA has plans to implement a sophisticated computer program that will search the Web for unauthorized disease treatment claims, potentially searching hundreds of thousands of Web sites per minute compared with a manual search by FDA staff, according to an FDA official. Moreover, although agency officials stated it was too early to determine the effectiveness of the newly established Current Good Manufacturing Practice regulations and serious adverse event reporting requirements, these new tools could improve the agency's ability to oversee the dietary supplement industry. While several stakeholders generally agreed that the new regulations could improve FDA's ability to oversee the dietary supplement industry, some stakeholders raised concerns about FDA's ability to enforce the new requirements given its limited resources.

Several Factors Limit FDA's Ability to Identify and Act on Safety Concerns Related to Dietary Supplements

Although FDA has taken some steps to identify and act on safety concerns, limited information hinders FDA's oversight of the dietary supplement industry. In addition, FDA dedicates relatively few resources to dietary supplement oversight. Furthermore, FDA is limited by a lack of authority to efficiently and effectively remove products from the market.

FDA's Ability to Identify Safety Concerns Is Hindered by a Lack of Information

FDA's ability to identify safety concerns is hindered by a lack of information in three key areas: the identity and location of dietary supplement firms; the types and contents of products on the market; and product safety information, such as adverse event data. First, FDA lacks complete information on the names and location of dietary supplement firms within the agency's jurisdiction. Although all dietary supplement firms must register with FDA as food facilities to provide information on their name and location, firms specializing in certain product categories, such as herbal products, are not required to self-identify as dietary supplement firms under current law. For example, a firm manufacturing products containing only herbs, such as echinacea and ginseng, would not be required to identify itself as a dietary supplement firm during the registration process. Consequently, FDA may not be aware of all dietary supplement firms that are currently operating. In addition, there is little assurance that FDA's existing inventory of dietary supplement firms is accurate because this information is not updated in a systematic fashion. As one FDA official explained, a thorough review of FDA's firm inventory would probably require dedicating 10 to 15 staff within each field office to the task for a year—which is unlikely given FDA's current workload. However, FDA officials did indicate that modifying the existing registration categories to better reflect FDA's inspection responsibilities could provide the agency with more complete information on the number and location of dietary supplement firms within its regulatory jurisdiction, provided industry complies with the new requirements. In FDA's *Food Protection Plan*, the agency requested statutory changes to allow modifying existing registration categories and require biannual renewals for food facilities, stating that such changes would ensure FDA has accurate, up-to-date information and would help the agency assess and respond to potential threats to the food supply.

Second, FDA does not have comprehensive information on the types and contents of dietary supplement products that are on the market or their ingredients. In addition, FDA officials noted that, if a dietary supplement firm reformulates a product to include different ingredients and/or changes the amounts of the ingredients without renaming the product, FDA may not be aware of the changes. Although drug manufacturers are required by law, with some exceptions, to register the identity and active ingredients of their products with FDA, the agency lacks the authority to require similar product information from dietary supplement manufacturers. Detailed product information could help the agency more efficiently and effectively analyze the adverse event reports it receives. For example, according to FDA, voluntary reports often contain inaccurate or incomplete information on product ingredients. Complete information on product ingredients could help the agency establish links between mandatory and voluntary reports on products containing the same ingredient. Furthermore, a database of marketed products and their ingredients could help the agency respond more quickly to safety concerns. For .instance, if FDA identified a particular ingredient of concern, officials could quickly determine which products on the market contained the ingredient and tailor the agency's response accordingly.

Third, FDA's ability to identify safety concerns is undermined by a lack of information on product safety, such as data on the frequency and characteristics of adverse events related to dietary supplements. As we noted earlier in this report, although dietary supplement firms are required to report all serious adverse event reports they have received to FDA, they are not required to report mild or moderate adverse events.[6] Additional information on adverse events could be particularly beneficial because there is a limited amount of scientific data available on the safety of dietary supplements compared with other regulated products such as drugs, which require premarket approval. For instance, FDA officials noted that mandatory reporting of mild and moderate events could assist the agency by increasing the amount of data available for signal detection, as well as provide additional support for safety-related conclusions regarding particular products or ingredients. Although some stakeholders have pointed out that mandatory manufacturer reporting of mild and moderate events won't fully address the issue of underreporting—particularly for consumers and health care providers—most medical researchers we interviewed agreed that mandatory reporting of all adverse events would be beneficial to the agency.

FDA Dedicates Relatively Few Resources to Dietary Supplement Oversight

FDA dedicates relatively few resources to dietary supplement oversight activities, including conducting inspections and developing guidance for industry on key safety-related aspects of DSHEA. Our analysis of FDA expenditure data found that FDA dedicated approximately 4 percent of CFSAN resources and 1 percent of its field resources—which are dedicated to FDA's Office of Regulatory Affairs—to dietary supplement programs from fiscal years 2006 through 2007.[7] FDA uses its field Dietary Supplements resources to, for example, monitor industry compliance by conducting surveillance actions such as inspections and import screenings. As FDA officials explained, limited inspection resources are prioritized according to public health risk, and dietary supplements are generally considered to be a lesser risk than, for example, foods that could be contaminated with foodborne pathogens. Consequently, although FDA conducted 973 inspections of foreign food firms from fiscal year 2002 through fiscal year 2008, FDA conducted no foreign inspections of dietary supplement firms during this time period.[8] Similarly, although FDA increased the number of domestic inspections of dietary supplement firms in fiscal years 2004 and 2005, overall, these inspections represented less than 1 percent of total food establishment inspections conducted by FDA and its state partners from fiscal years 2002 through 2008. With few resources dedicated to dietary supplement inspections, FDA's ability to identify potential safety concerns through this key surveillance activity is limited.

Furthermore, despite identifying the need to provide industry with guidance on key aspects of DSHEA, FDA has not done so in a timely manner. For example, DSHEA authorized FDA to establish Current Good Manufacturing Practices specific to dietary supplements in 1994; however, the agency did not publish a proposed rule until 2003 and did not finalize the rule until 2007. FDA officials noted that it first issued an advance notice of proposed rulemaking in 1997 and went through a number of steps, such as conducting public meetings, to develop an overall strategy for regulating dietary supplements and then submitted its rule to the Office of Management and Budget for clearance before finalizing the rule. Because these Current Good Manufacturing Practices are phased in over time, they will not fully be in effect until 2010—16 years after FDA was authorized to establish them.

In addition, although FDA recognized the need to develop guidance on the new dietary ingredient provisions of DSHEA, FDA has yet to issue this guidance—an omission previously highlighted in our 2000 report. As an FDA official explained, new dietary ingredient guidance is critical for dietary supplement safety because, without formal guidance, firms may not notify FDA before marketing products that have drastically different safety profiles than their historical use. For example, this official was concerned that a firm could use bitter orange's historical use as a flavoring in marmalade as justification for not submitting a new dietary ingredient notification to FDA when it uses bitter orange to create a product that is 95 percent synephrine—a powerful stimulant. Similarly, a firm might choose to market dietary supplement products that contain nano-sized particles of grandfathered ingredients without notifying FDA in advance. According to the FDA official, this raises concerns because potential health risks associated with nano-sized particles are unknown. According to this official, FDA has started to develop draft guidance for new dietary ingredients that would clarify what factors FDA will use when determining if a substance is a new dietary ingredient. More specifically, the guidance would clarify what changes to grandfathered ingredients would require a new dietary ingredient notification to FDA and what information should be included in the notification, among other items. However, this draft guidance has been under legal review for over a year, and FDA did not provide us with a time frame for its issuance.

FDA's Lack of Authority Limits Its Ability to Remove Products from the Market

Once FDA has identified a safety concern, the agency's ability to efficiently and effectively remove a product from the market is hindered by a lack of mandatory recall authority. For instance, FDA officials commented that FDA's ability to protect consumers through its voluntary recall authority is limited because it relies on industry exercising its responsibility rather than enforceable requirements. As FDA noted in its *Food Protection Plan*, mandatory recall authority would allow the agency to ensure the prompt and complete removal of unsafe products from distribution channels in cases where a firm was unwilling to cooperate voluntarily.

Additionally, agency officials and other stakeholders have acknowledged the difficulty of banning a dietary supplement because FDA must establish adulteration under the significant or unreasonable risk standard. For example, it took FDA almost 10 years after issuing its first advisory about ephedra to gather sufficient data to meet the statutory burden of proof for banning ephedra from the market. The difficulty of establishing significant or unreasonable risk is compounded by limited scientific research on the safety of dietary supplements—

which are generally presumed safe under the law, and firms are not required to provide FDA with evidence of product safety for ingredients marketed prior to October 15, 1994, such as ephedra. Underreporting of adverse events also limits FDA's ability to meet its burden of proof. In the case of ephedra, one firm withheld information from FDA on thousands of serious adverse event reports related to its product—which hindered FDA's investigation, and prompted support for establishing mandatory reporting requirements. As previously mentioned in this report, although mandatory serious adverse event reporting requirements for industry are now in effect, underreporting of all adverse events from consumers, health care providers, and industry remains a concern. According to an agency official, given these data limitations and the agency's difficult and costly experience with ephedra, banning an ingredient is not a very viable option. However, according to some experts, the difficult process of establishing significant or unreasonable risk for dietary supplement ingredients with known safety concerns has raised doubts about FDA's ability to adequately protect the public. For example, table 5 summarizes FDA actions for certain dietary supplement ingredients that have been banned in other countries.

Table 5. Examples of FDA Actions Taken on Dietary Supplement Ingredients That Have Been Banned in Other Countries

Ingredient	Reported uses	Dangers	Regulatory actionns in other countries	FDA actions
Aristolochic acid	Aphrodisiac, immune stimulant	Kidney damage, cancers, deaths reported.	Banned in seven European countries, Japan, Venezuela, and Egypt.	In 2000 and 2001, FDA listed aristolochic acid as a "Botanical Ingredient of Concern" and issued letters to industry and health care professionals. In 2001, FDA issued an "Import Alert" for products containing the ingredient and issued a consumer advisory. FDA has also taken some enforcement or advisory actions against individual products.
Kava	Anxiety, stress	Abnormal liver function or damage, deaths	Banned in Canada, Germany, Singapore, South	FDA issued letters to health care professionals in 2001 and 2002 and a consumer advisory in 2002.

		reported.	Africa, and Switzerland.	
Lobelia	Asthma, bronchitis	Tremor, overdose may cause coma and possibly death.	Banned in Bangladesh and Italy.	No action.

Source: GAO analysis of FDA and Consumer's Union data.
Note: GAO did not independently verify regulatory actions in other countries.

WHILE FDA HAS TAKEN SOME ACTIONS WHEN FOODS CONTAIN UNSAFE DIETARY INGREDIENTS, CERTAIN FACTORS MAY ALLOW UNSAFE PRODUCTS TO REACH CONSUMERS

Although FDA has taken some actions, such as issuing warnings, when foods contain unsafe dietary ingredients, certain factors may allow unsafe products to reach consumers. FDA may not know when a company has made an unsupported or incorrect GRAS determination about an added dietary ingredient in a product until after the product becomes available to consumers because companies are not required to notify FDA of their self-determinations. In addition, the boundary between dietary supplements and foods containing added dietary ingredients is not always clear, and some food products could be marketed as dietary supplements to circumvent the safety standard required for food additives. Finally, according to FDA officials, the agency conducts a limited amount of monitoring for safety concerns associated with foods containing added dietary ingredients.

Companies Are Not Required to Notify FDA When They Make a Self-Determination That an Added Ingredient Is GRAS

The Federal Food, Drug, and Cosmetic Act allows companies to market a conventional food product with added dietary ingredients if the company determines that the added dietary ingredient meets the GRAS standard. These companies do not have to notify FDA before selling the product to consumers, although some may do so voluntarily. If a company makes an unsupported or incorrect GRAS determination about an added dietary ingredient in a product, FDA may not know about the product until after it becomes available to consumers. This was the case, for example, for several food products containing such herbs as kava, ginkgo, and echinacea. Specific examples are as follows:

- In 2004, during a food inspection of a juice company, FDA found that the company was marketing a product that contained kava. According to FDA, it is not aware of a basis for concluding that kava is GRAS, and it has not approved kava as a food additive. In addition, kava was the subject of a public health advisory issued by FDA in March 2002, which warned consumers of the potential risk of severe liver injury associated with the use of kava.

- In 2001, FDA identified a company marketing cereals with ginkgo biloba and Siberian ginseng. According to FDA, it is not aware of a basis for concluding that these ingredients are GRAS, and it has not approved them as food additives. FDA sent a warning letter to the company, and the product was subsequently removed from the market.

- Also in 2001, FDA identified a company marketing juices with added echinacea. FDA sent a warning to the company noting that it has not approved echinacea as a food additive and is not aware of a basis for concluding that echinacea is GRAS.

FDA learned of these products after they were available to consumers. If FDA wanted to remove these products from the market, and the companies did not do so voluntarily, FDA would have to initiate enforcement actions.

The Boundary between Dietary Supplements and Foods with Added Dietary Ingredients Is Not Always Clear

The boundary between dietary supplements and foods containing added dietary ingredients is not always clear. FDA officials have noted, for example, that a tea with an identical mix of herbal ingredients could be considered either a dietary supplement or a food product. FDA determines how to classify the tea based on the product labeling. More specifically, according to FDA, if the tea is labeled as a dietary supplement and is not represented as a conventional food, FDA would consider the tea to be a dietary supplement and regulate it as such. On the other hand, if the tea is labeled as a food or is represented as a conventional food with terms such as "drink" or "beverage," FDA officials noted that they would consider the tea to be a food.

The way FDA classifies a product is important because the safety standard that applies to the product varies based on that classification. If the product is classified as a conventional food, the added dietary ingredient must meet the GRAS standard or be approved by FDA as a food additive, except in certain circumstances as authorized in law. If the product is classified as a dietary supplement, the added dietary ingredient is presumed safe if it was marketed in the United States before October 15, 1994; otherwise, it is considered a new dietary ingredient, and the manufacturer or distributor may be required to notify FDA 75 days before the product with the added dietary ingredient enters the market and provide some basis for concluding that the ingredient is reasonably expected to be safe. According to FDA and industry officials, this is a less stringent standard than that for food additives. However, FDA does not have the authority to require that the safety of dietary supplements be approved before entering the market.

These differences in how products are regulated may lead to circumstances when an ingredient would not be allowed to be added to a product if it was labeled as a conventional food but would be allowed in the identical product if it was labeled as a dietary supplement. This was the case, for example, in August 2007, when FDA identified a company marketing an iced tea mix containing stevia—an herb that had not been approved as a food additive because of potential safety concerns, including reproductive and cardiovascular effects. FDA issued a warning to the company; however, rather than discontinue using stevia in its product, the company changed the label to classify the product as a dietary supplement rather than a food, and the product remains on the market. We identified other products that also fall within the gray area between dietary supplements and foods with added dietary ingredients that are being marketed as dietary supplements. For example, we identified several nutrition bars, teas, and energy drinks, some produced by large companies with national distribution, which contain herbs such as kava, St. John's wort, and echinacea. If these ingredients are added to conventional foods and are not GRAS and have not been approved as food additives, then they would violate the Federal Food, Drug, and Cosmetic Act. An FDA official told us that FDA is unaware of a basis for concluding that these ingredients are GRAS, and they have not been approved as food additives. However, these products may remain on the market because they are labeled as dietary supplements. Such a process might allow companies to circumvent the safety standard required for food additives.

In FDA's 10-year plan to implement DSHEA, issued in January 2000, the agency identified the need to clarify the boundary between conventional foods and dietary supplements but did not indicate when or how the agency planned to address this issue. Moreover, we highlighted this particular issue in our July 2000 report and recommended FDA take action to clarify the boundary between conventional foods and dietary supplements. As of November 2008, the agency had not issued regulations or guidance to clarify this boundary.

FDA Conducts Limited Monitoring of Foods with Added Dietary Ingredients

According to FDA officials, the agency conducts limited monitoring for safety concerns associated with food products that contain added dietary ingredients. These officials explained that FDA does not track these products separately from foods, and the agency generally relies on trade complaints and adverse event reports to identify concerns about these types of products. FDA officials told us that the current regulatory framework is sufficient to identify and act on safety concerns regarding foods with added dietary ingredients. FDA held a public meeting in 2006 regarding these products and, according to FDA officials, the agency is currently evaluating the comments made during that meeting.

Some stakeholders told us that safety risks associated with foods containing added dietary ingredients that meet the GRAS standard or have been approved as food additives are generally low. For example, stakeholders were generally not concerned about vitamin-fortified products, such as cereal, unless individuals consume these products in high doses. However, some stakeholders we spoke with raised concerns about certain products—such as energy drinks that contain stimulants and have the potential to cause adverse cardiac effects. In addition, some stakeholders expressed concern about adding botanicals to foods due, in part, to the potential for an adverse physiological response. In contrast, an industry official noted that companies sometimes add dietary ingredients to foods for labeling or marketing purposes—not to elicit a physiological effect—and, therefore, the amounts included are low.

FDA HAS TAKEN LIMITED STEPS TO EDUCATE CONSUMERS ABOUT DIETARY SUPPLEMENTS, AND CONSUMERS REMAIN LARGELY UNINFORMED

While FDA has conducted some consumer outreach, these initiatives have reached a relatively small proportion of consumers using dietary supplements.

Additionally, surveys and experts indicate that consumers are not well-informed about the safety and efficacy of dietary supplements and have difficulty interpreting labels on these products. Without a clear understanding of the safety, efficacy, and labeling of dietary supplements, consumers may be exposed to greater health risks associated with the uninformed use of these products.

FDA Has Conducted Some Consumer Education about Dietary Supplements, but These Efforts Have Been Limited

FDA has taken some steps to educate consumers about the safety, efficacy, and labeling of dietary supplements. According to FDA officials, the agency primarily educates the public about dietary supplements through publications such as brochures and articles, as well as the agency's Web site. For example, agency officials highlighted the following efforts:

- FDA and the NIH's Office of Dietary Supplements jointly published a brochure in 2004 to educate consumers about the importance of disclosing their dietary supplement usage to doctors.
- In March 2006, FDA developed a document entitled, "Food Facts: Dietary Supplements—What You Need to Know" with general information about dietary supplements.
- In August 2008, FDA distributed an article via e-mail and its Web site entitled "FDA 101: Dietary Supplements" that contained information on the regulation of dietary supplements, as well as information on the safety, efficacy, and labeling of these products.
- FDA's Web site provides warnings about certain ingredients and products, how to report an adverse event, and general consumer information about dietary supplements, including descriptions of the types of label claims permitted on dietary supplement products. FDA's Web site also links consumers to the NIH, Federal Trade Commission, United States Department of Agriculture, and National Academies' Institute of Medicine Web pages that contain information about the safety and efficacy of certain dietary supplement ingredients and how to interpret dietary supplement labels.
- FDA has worked jointly with industry, consumer groups, and other federal agencies to provide consumers with information about label claims.

However, these outreach efforts can only be as effective as the number of dietary supplement users they reach. While data from the 2007 National Health Interview Survey show that over half of the U.S. adult population—or at least 114 million individuals—consume dietary supplements, we found that FDA's outreach efforts have limited potential to reach the majority of U.S. adults using dietary supplements. For example, according to FDA and NIH officials, since 2004, the brochure regarding disclosure of supplement use to doctors had a distribution of 40,000 paper copies and received about 171,000 total visits on the FDA and NIH Web sites—which represent less than 1 percent of estimated dietary supplement users. Other FDA publications on dietary supplements have also reached a relatively small proportion of dietary supplement consumers. For example, according to FDA officials, it distributed about 61,000 English copies and approximately 35,000 Spanish copies of its document entitled "Food Facts: Dietary Supplements—What You Need to Know." In addition, according to FDA officials, its consumer article on dietary supplements called "FDA 101: Dietary Supplements" was sent via e-mail to almost 32,500 subscribers to FDA's "Consumer Health Information" and, as of October 21, 2008, FDA's Web site had logged about 3,800 page views of the HTML version and approximately 2,100 page views of the printer-friendly PDF of the article.

While agency officials stated that FDA does not evaluate the effectiveness of its outreach efforts, officials also noted that the agency must continually market its desired messages to effectively educate consumers.

Additionally, consumer education was highlighted as an important part of the agency's 10-year plan for dietary supplements, published in 2000. In the November 2004 update to this plan, FDA identified the need to provide consumers with access to reliable scientific information about the safety of ingredients and supplements so that consumers may make more informed choices. Currently, according to FDA, CFSAN has no ongoing or new consumer education initiatives being planned for dietary supplements. FDA recently announced a partnership with WebMD to expand consumer access to timely and reliable health information; however, it is not clear to what extent FDA will use this partnership to increase consumer understanding about dietary supplements. When asked about plans for consumer education initiatives, FDA officials explained that the agency has been directing its limited resources toward activities that can have the greatest public health impact, such as responding to foodborne illness outbreaks.

Consumers Are Not Well-Informed about the Safety, Efficacy, and Labeling of Dietary Supplements

Several studies indicate that consumers are not well-informed about the safety, efficacy, and labeling of dietary supplements. For example, a 2002 Harris Poll indicated that a majority of adults are misinformed about the extent to which government regulates the safety of vitamins, minerals, and food supplements. According to the poll, over half of respondents believed that dietary supplements are approved by a government agency. A 2002 FDA-sponsored health and diet survey also estimated that a majority of respondents who used vitamin or mineral supplements believed that the government approves dietary supplement products before they are marketed to consumers. However, FDA does not have the authority to require that supplements be approved for safety and effectiveness prior to marketing, and, unless a product contains a new dietary ingredient, FDA does not need to be notified by the manufacturer prior to marketing a dietary supplement. Additionally, the 2002 Harris Poll estimated that about two-thirds of respondents believe that the government requires dietary supplement labels to contain warnings about potential side effects, or dangers, similar to drugs. However, unlike drug manufacturers, who are required to include warnings related to adverse effects and contraindications on their product labels, dietary supplement manufacturers are required to include few such warnings on their product labels. Consequently, dietary supplement manufacturers may not necessarily include warnings about potential adverse effects on the labels of their products. For example, in the course of our review, we identified several dietary supplements that contained ingredients with known or suspected adverse effects, such as kava and black cohosh, that did not include warnings on their labels. In addition, in 2003, an analysis of 100 dietary supplement labels by the Department of Health and Human Services' Office of Inspector General found that the dietary supplement labels were limited in their ability to guide the informed and appropriate use of dietary supplements among consumers and often did not present information in a manner that facilitates consumer understanding.[9]

Furthermore, during the course of our review, most experts we spoke with noted that, generally, consumers are not well-informed about the safety and efficacy of dietary supplements. These experts explained that many consumers believe various myths about dietary supplements. For example, consumers may believe that if a product is natural, it must be safe; if a little is good, then more must be better; and if a product does not have a warning label, it must be safe. Without a clear understanding of the safety, efficacy, and labeling of dietary supplements, consumers are exposed to potential health risks associated with the uninformed use of these products. For example, several experts stated that misconceptions about dietary supplements could cause consumers to incorrectly assess the risks and benefits of these products and, in some cases, substitute supplements for prescribed medicine. In addition, several experts noted that consumers may not be aware that taking combinations of some supplements or using certain products in conjunction with prescription drugs could lead to harmful and potentially life-threatening results. In particular, some supplements—such as garlic, ginkgo biloba, ginseng, and vitamin E—may cause blood thinning and lead to life-threatening complications during surgical procedures. Therefore, consumer education is critical to mitigate the potential risks associated with the uninformed use of dietary supplements.

CONCLUSIONS

Americans are widely interested in maintaining health and wellness and, with an aging population, we expect that consumers' interest in dietary supplements will continue to grow. These consumers confront an extensive variety of dietary supplements available in the marketplace, but little is known about the safety and efficacy of these products. Yet, most dietary supplements are presumed safe under current law, and companies do not need premarket approval for any dietary supplement. If FDA has concerns about a particular dietary supplement product or ingredient, the agency bears the burden of proof to require removal of the product from the market. In the case of ephedra—which was implicated in thousands of adverse events and a number of deaths—FDA faced a long and arduous process before finally banning the product in 2004.

At the same time, while more and more products are entering the market each year, FDA is dedicating a small percentage of its resources to regulating the dietary supplement industry and educating consumers about dietary supplements. FDA does not have comprehensive knowledge of dietary supplement manufacturers or the products on the market and has little information about potential side effects of various products. In addition, consumers are not well-informed about dietary supplements, may not be aware of potential side effects of supplements, and might not consider a dietary supplement as a factor if experiencing an adverse reaction. Weaknesses in the regulatory system may increase the likelihood of unsafe products reaching the market, and a lack of consumer knowledge increases the potential health risks associated with uninformed consumption.

RECOMMENDATIONS FOR EXECUTIVE ACTION

Overall, we are making four recommendations to enhance FDA's oversight of dietary supplements and foods with added dietary ingredients.

To improve the information available to FDA for identifying safety concerns and better enable FDA to meet its responsibility to protect the public health, we recommend that the Secretary of the Department of Health and Human Services direct the Commissioner of FDA to request authority to require dietary supplement companies to

- identify themselves as a dietary supplement company as part of the existing registration requirements and update this information annually,
- provide a list of all dietary supplement products they sell and a copy of the labels and update this information annually, and
- report all adverse events related to dietary supplements.

To better enable FDA to meet its responsibility to regulate dietary supplements that contain new dietary ingredients, we recommend that the Secretary of the Department of Health and Human Services direct the Commissioner of FDA to issue guidance to clarify when an ingredient is considered a new dietary ingredient, the evidence needed to document the safety of new dietary ingredients, and appropriate methods for establishing ingredient identity.

To help ensure that companies follow the appropriate laws and regulations and to renew a recommendation we made in July 2000, we recommend that the Secretary of the Department of Health and Human Services direct the Commissioner of FDA to provide guidance to industry to clarify when products should be marketed as either dietary supplements or conventional foods formulated with added dietary ingredients.

To improve consumer understanding about dietary supplements and better leverage existing resources, we recommend that the Secretary of the Department of Health and Human Services direct the Commissioner of FDA to coordinate with stakeholder groups involved in consumer outreach to (1) identify additional mechanisms—such as the recent WebMD partnership—for educating consumers about the safety, efficacy, and labeling of dietary supplements; (2) implement these mechanisms; and (3) assess their effectiveness.

AGENCY COMMENTS AND OUR EVALUATION

We provided a draft copy of this report to the Department of Health and Human Services for review and comment. We received a written response from the Acting Assistant Secretary for Legislation that included comments from FDA. FDA generally agreed with each of the report's recommendations and welcomed the report as a means of calling attention to the challenges FDA faces with respect to regulating dietary supplements and conventional foods formulated with added dietary ingredients. FDA noted that although receiving information on all adverse events related to dietary supplements could enhance FDA's ability to detect signals of potential toxicity over time, FDA raised concerns about its ability to efficiently and effectively analyze the information to identify unsafe dietary supplements. However, FDA stated that it is working on methodologies to mitigate this concern and improve data mining for safety-related signals if FDA were to receive all adverse event reports. In addition, FDA recognized the need for guidance to industry clarifying when products should be marketed as conventional foods or dietary supplements and stated that the agency will consider this recommendation and its implementation in light of FDA's limited resources and competing priorities. Furthermore, FDA noted that the agency's resources for consumer education are extremely limited and that it may not be able to effectively conduct consumer education on its own. FDA commented that collaborating with NIH's Office of Dietary Supplements may be an efficient and cost-effective way to expand FDA's current outreach activities. FDA also stated that the agency is identifying appropriate content for the recently announced FDA/WebMD partnership referenced in the report and anticipates that information on dietary supplements will be included. FDA's comments are presented in appendix IV of this report. FDA also provided technical comments on the draft report, which we incorporated as appropriate.

As agreed with your offices, unless you publicly announce the contents of this report earlier, we plan no further distribution until 30 days from the report date. At that time, we will send copies to the appropriate congressional committees; the Secretary of the Department of Health and Human Services; the Commissioner of FDA; the Director of the Office of Management and Budget; and other interested parties. The report also will be available at no charge on the GAO Web site at http://www.gao.gov.

If you or your staffs have any questions about this report, please contact me at (202) 512-3841 or shamesl@gao.gov. Contact points for our Offices of Congressional Relations and Public Affairs may be found on the last page of this report. GAO staff who made major contributions to this report are listed in appendix V.

Lisa Shames
Director, Natural Resources and Environment

APPENDIX I: OBJECTIVES, SCOPE, AND METHODOLOGY

We were asked to examine the Food and Drug Administration's (FDA) oversight of dietary supplements and foods that contain added dietary ingredients. Specifically, we were asked to examine FDA's (1) actions to respond to the new serious adverse event reporting requirements; (2) ability to identify and act on concerns about the safety of dietary supplements; (3) ability to identify and act on concerns about the safety of foods with added dietary ingredients; and (4) actions to educate consumers about the safety, efficacy, and labeling of dietary supplements. Our work included dietary supplements for human use only. We did not assess FDA's regulation of dietary supplements for animal use.

To identify FDA's actions to respond to the new serious adverse event reporting requirements, we reviewed FDA's guidance on reporting requirements for industry and internal procedures for compiling and tracking adverse event reports. In addition, we obtained and analyzed data on the number and type of reports received before and after the requirements went into effect. We verified our methodology for analyzing these data with FDA officials, and FDA verified our results. We also reviewed FDA's plans for improving adverse event reporting.

To examine FDA's ability to identify and act on safety concerns associated with dietary supplements, we assessed FDA's laws, rules, regulations, planning documents and guidance, such as the Dietary Supplement Health and Education Act of 1994, Current Good Manufacturing Practice regulations, and guidance on reporting adverse events. In addition, we obtained and analyzed data on FDA's internal procedures and activities to identify safety concerns, such as conducting inspections and import screenings and receiving consumer complaints. We also obtained and analyzed FDA's internal procedures and data on the agency's actions once a safety concern is identified, including issuing warning letters, seizing products, and banning ingredients. We analyzed these data to determine the range and extent of actions FDA has taken to identify and act on safety concerns associated with dietary supplements. We verified our methodology for analyzing these data with FDA officials, and FDA verified our results. Furthermore, we reviewed data on FDA resources dedicated to dietary supplements.

To examine FDA's ability to identify and act on concerns about the safety of foods with added dietary ingredients, we reviewed laws and regulations regarding food additives. In addition, we reviewed FDA's procedures for identifying and acting on safety concerns of foods with added dietary ingredients. We also identified and analyzed instances of actions taken by FDA to act on safety concerns associated with the addition of dietary ingredients to foods.

To determine FDA's actions to educate consumers about the safety, efficacy, and labeling of dietary supplements, we reviewed FDA's consumer outreach initiatives. We also obtained and analyzed data on the extent to which these outreach initiatives were distributed. In addition, we analyzed data from FDA and others on consumer understanding of dietary supplements.

To compare FDA's regulation of dietary supplements with select other countries' regulation of these products, we spoke with representatives from the governments of Canada, Japan, and the United Kingdom. In addition, we reviewed documents about the regulation of dietary supplements in these countries. We did not independently verify descriptions of foreign laws. We selected these countries because they had been identified in prior GAO work as having comparable food safety systems and covered a relatively diverse geographic area (Europe, North America, and Asia.)

To assess the reliability of the data from FDA's databases used in this report, we reviewed related documentation, examined the data to identify obvious errors or inconsistencies, and worked with agency officials to identify any data problems. We determined the data to be sufficiently reliable for the purposes of this report.

To obtain insights on all four objectives, we met with a wide range of experts, including officials from federal and state agencies, industry and trade organizations, consumer advocacy groups, academia, and poison control centers. Through these efforts, we obtained documents and information related to all four objectives. At the federal level, we met with officials from FDA, including headquarters and regional and district level officials, to discuss the agency's regulatory authorities, actions taken to implement the mandatory adverse event reporting system, steps taken to regulate the safety of dietary supplements and foods with added dietary ingredients, and consumer education responsibilities and actions. In addition, we met with officials from the National Institutes of Health, Federal Trade Commission, and Department of Agriculture. At the state level, we met with officials from the California Department of Public Health's Food and Drug Branch and Environmental Protection Agency and the New York State Task Force on Life and the Law. To obtain insights from the dietary supplement and food industries, we met with officials from the American Beverage Association, American Herbal Products Association, Consumer Healthcare Products Association, Council for Responsible Nutrition, Grocery Manufacturers Association, National Advertising Division of the Council of Better Business Bureaus, and Natural Products Association. In addition, we met with officials from a large dietary supplement manufacturer in Maryland, a multinational food and consumer products firm, and two small, herbal products manufacturers in

California. To obtain insights from consumer advocacy groups, we met with officials from the Center for Science in the Public Interest, Consumers Union, and Public Citizen. To obtain insights from public health organizations, the health care community, and academia, we met with officials from the American Association of Poison Control Centers; American Medical Association; California Poison Control System; New York City Poison Control Center; U.S. Pharmacopoeia; Baylor College of Medicine; Critical Path Institute; Center for Advanced Food Technology, Rutgers University; Stony Brook University; Center for Consumer Self Care, Department of Clinical Pharmacy, and Osher Center for Integrative Medicine, University of California, San Francisco; and the University of California, Berkeley.

We conducted this performance audit from December 2007 through January 2009, in accordance with generally accepted government auditing standards. Those standards require that we plan and perform the audit to obtain sufficient, appropriate evidence to provide a reasonable basis for our findings and conclusions based on our audit objectives. We believe that the evidence obtained provides a reasonable basis for our findings and conclusions based on our audit objectives.

APPENDIX II: DATA ON FDA'S ACTIONS TO IDENTIFY AND RESPOND TO SAFETY CONCERNS RELATED TO DIETARY SUPPLEMENTS

This appendix provides additional detail on FDA's actions to identify and respond to safety concerns related to dietary supplements.

Data on FDA's Actions to Identify Safety Concerns Related to Dietary Supplements

FDA actions to identify safety concerns related to dietary supplements include receiving and analyzing adverse event reports and consumer complaints and conducting inspections.

Table 6. Comparison of the Number of Adverse Event Reports Received and Entered into FDA's Databases for Review Related to Dietary Supplements and Drugs and Biologics, January 1, 2003, through December 31, 2007

Description	Year					Total Average	
	2003	2004	2005	2006	2007		
Total dietary supplement reports received and entered for review	739	657	491	317	350	2,554	511
Total drugs and biologics reports received and entered for review	226,217	273,601	323,384	337,155	364,449	1,524,806	304,961

Source: GAO analysis of FDA data.

Notes: Dietary Supplement Reports includes both voluntary and mandatory adverse event reports. If a report is incomplete, it is not entered into the report database. FDA receives roughly 30 incomplete reports related to dietary supplements per month. According to FDA, reporting rates were higher in 2003 and 2004 due to adverse events related to ephedra. FDA requires firms to report serious and nonserious adverse events for new drugs.

Data on Adverse Events Related to Dietary Supplements

Table 6 compares the number of adverse event reports received and entered into FDA's databases for review related to dietary supplements and drugs and biologics from January 1, 2003, through December 31, 2007.

Table 7 compares the number of dietary supplement-related adverse event cases characterized as serious from January 1, 2003, through October 31, 2008, and the total number of dietary supplement-related adverse event cases.

Table 7. Number of Dietary Supplement-Related Adverse Event Cases Characterized as Serious, January 1, 2003, through October 31, 2008

Description	Year						Total
	2003	2004	2005	2006	2007	2008	
Cases characterized as serious	510[a]	483	364	213	213	759	2,542
Total number of dietary supplement-related cases	**739**	**657**	**491**	**317**	**350**	**948**	**3,502**

Source: FDA.

[a] Thirty-six reports did not contain information about seriousness in 2003.

Table 8 shows the number and types of outcomes for all dietary supplement-related adverse event cases received by FDA from January 1, 2003, through October 31, 2008.

Table 8. Number of Dietary Supplement-Related Adverse Event Complaint (AEC) Outcomes for all Adverse Event Cases, January 1, 2003, through October 31, 2008

Description	Year							Percentage of dietary supplement-related cases
	2003	2004	2005	2006	2007	2008	Total	
Hospitalization	245	217	165	86	93	301	**1,107**	31.6%
Nonserious injuries / illness	310	259	149	72	77	109	**976**	27.9
Serious injuries / illness	35	100	113	38	43	540	**869**	24.8
Visited a health care provider	200	171	100	81	97	218	**867**	24.8

Description	Year							Percentage of dietary supplement-related cases
	2003	2004	2005	2006	2007	2008	Total	
Other serious (important medical events)	0	0	13	92	99	407	**611**	17.4
Visited an emergency room	114	98	78	44	52	152	**538**	15.4
Life-threatening	89	108	51	41	64	118	**471**	13.4
Requires intervention to prevent permanent impairment	82	127	68	24	28	40	**369**	10.5
Death	52	35	26	11	7	11	**142**	4.1
Disability	33	37	14	17	14	19	**134**	3.8
Other	13	3	3	0	0	0	**19**	0.5
Congenital anomaly	2	3	1	0	2	0	**8**	0.2%
Total number of cases with AEC outcome[a]	**739**	**657**	**491**	**317**	**350**	**948**	**3,502**	

Source: FDA.

[a] Cases may have more than one adverse event reported outcome; therefore, the sum of outcomes exceeds the total number of cases per year.

Table 9 shows the number of dietary supplement-related adverse event cases by product type from January 1, 2003, through October 31, 2008.

Table 9. Number of All Dietary Supplement-Related Cases with Reported Adverse Event Outcomes by Product Classification, January 1, 2003, through October 31, 2008

Product classification	Cases	Percentage of dietary supplement-related cases
Combination products and products not elsewhere classified	1,566	44.7%
Herbal and botanical (other than teas)	1,017	29.0
Vitamin	658	18.8
Mineral	373	10.7
Fats and lipid substances	108	3.1

Table 9. (Continued)

Product classification	Cases	Percentage of dietary suppl-ement-related cases
Herbal and botanical teas	92	2.6
Protein	78	2.2
Fiber	53	1.5
Unknown	14	0.4
Animal by-products and extracts	11	0.3%
Total number of cases[a]	**3,502**	

Source: FDA.

[a] Cases may have more than one product classification; therefore, the sum of cases by product classification may exceed the total number of cases.

Data on Consumer Complaints Related to Dietary Supplements

Table 10 shows the number of dietary supplement-related consumer complaints by adverse event result for fiscal year 2001 through July 3, 2008.

Table 10. Number of Dietary Supplement-Related Consumer Complaints by Adverse Event Result, Fiscal Year 2001 through July 3, 2008

Description	Year								Total	Percentage of total dietary supplement-related consumer complaints
	2001	2002	2003	2004	2005	2006	2007	2008		
No adverse events or symptoms reported[a]	111	98	81	69	64	60	50	53	**586**	57.6%
Nonlife-threatening illness	39	23	31	14	9	12	21	20	**169**	16.6
Nonlife-threatening—no adverse event reporting (adverse symptoms present)[b]	10	20	25	20	17	22	27	23	**164**	16.1

Description	Year								Total	Percentage of total dietary supplement-related consumer complaints
	2001	2002	2003	2004	2005	2006	2007	2008		
Life-threatening illness	19	8	27	10	3	2	10	6	**85**	8.3
Death	1	2	4	2	2	2	1	0	**14**	1.4
Total									**1018**	**100.0%**

Source: GAO analysis of FDA data.

Note: FDA pulled these data from its FACTS database. These data are a subset of the data provided in table 9. At the time the complaint is entered into FACTS, there is no verification that a death, illness, or injury was a direct consequence of the dietary supplement consumed.

[a] This category includes complaints where the adverse event result was "None," blank, or "Nonlife-threatening—no adverse event reporting" when there were no adverse symptoms present.

[b] According to an FDA official, "Nonlife-threatening—no adverse event reporting" does not mean that an adverse event is not present; rather, this category is selected by field staff when they do not have enough information initially to fill all of the required fields in the adverse event reporting screen within FDA's database for consumer complaints.

Table 11 shows the number of dietary supplement-related consumer complaints with adverse symptoms present by adverse event result and FDA product class from fiscal year 2001 through July 3, 2008.

Data on Inspections Related to Dietary Supplements

Table 12 shows the number of foreign and domestic inspections of dietary supplement facilities compared with food inspections and total inspections conducted by FDA and states from fiscal years 2000 through 2008.

Table 13 shows the percentage of dietary supplement inspections where investigators identified problems, from fiscal year 2002 through May 6, 2008.

Table 11. Number of Dietary Supplement-Related Consumer Complaints with Adverse Symptoms Present by Adverse Event Result and Product Classification, Fiscal Year 2001 through July 3, 2008

Description	FDA product classification									Total
	Herbal and botanical (other than teas)	Animal by-products and extracts	Herbal and botanical teas	Combination products and products not else-where classified	Vitamin	Mineral	Protein	Fats and lipid substances	Other (all other classes)	
Death	8	1	1	3	1	0	0	0	0	14
Life-threatening illness	40	0	3	26	5	4	2	1	4	85
Nonlife-threatening illness	48	1	5	72	14	8	11	3	7	169
Nonlife-threatening—no adverse event reporting (adverse symptoms present)[a]	43	1	7	54	21	14	11	6	7	164
Total in product class for complaints with adverse events or systems reported	**139**	**3**	**16**	**155**	**41**	**26**	**24**	**10**	**18**	**432**
Percentage of total product classes for complaints with adverse events or symptoms reported	32.2%	0.7%	3.7%	35.9%	9.5%	6.0%	5.6%	2.3%	4.2%	100.0%

Source: GAO analysis of FDA data.

Note: FDA pulled these data from its FACTS database. These data are a subset of the data provided in table 9. At the time the complaint is entered into FACTS, there is no verification that a death, illness, or injury was a direct consequence of the dietary supplement consumed.

[a] According to an FDA official, "Nonlife-threatening—no adverse event reporting" does not mean that an adverse event isn't present; rather, this category is selected by field staff when they do not have enough information initially to fill all of the required fields in the adverse event reporting screen within FDA's database for consumer complaints.

Table 12. FDA Foreign and Domestic Inspections and State Domestic Inspections, Fiscal Years 2000 through 2008

Description	Fiscal year									Total
	2000	2001	2002	2003	2004	2005	2006	2007	2008	
FDA foreign										
Dietary supplement inspections[a]	0	0	0	0	0	0	0	0	0	0
Foods inspections	177	211	169	148	153	132	125	96	150	1,361
All FDA inspections	878	892	791	757	932	844	789	1,005	933	7,821
FDA domestic										
Dietary supplement inspections[a]	60	71	66	87	163	167	137	119	65	935
Foods inspections	6,728	9,811	8,742	11,295	11,013	8,775	7,510	6,500	6,559	76,933
All FDA inspections	14,257	17,785	17,854	21,812	20,898	19,013	16,869	14,623	14,328	157,439
State domestic										
Dietary supplement inspections[a, b]	0	0	4	1	33	39	18	9	1	105
Foods inspections	6,546	7,667	7,921	8,252	8,763	9,388	8,918	9,751	9,183	76,389
All state inspections	16,312	18,078	21,160	20,625	21,894	22,381	23,935	25,146	23,373	192,904

Source: FDA.

Note: Food inspections, all FDA inspections, and all state inspections categories include dietary supplement inspections that were conducted during the designated time period.

[a] Dietary supplement inspections excludes those inspections related to dietary supplements with drug or veterinary uses. Data is current as of November 19, 2008. Because FDA's inspection database is continuously updated, these numbers may change as state and district offices enter new information or existing information is corrected.

[b] According to an FDA official, dietary supplement inspections conducted by states during this time period were performed under a partnership agreement rather than a FDA contract.

Table 13. Share of Dietary Supplement Inspections Where Investigators Identified Problems, Fiscal Year 2002 through May 6, 2008[a]

Description	Fiscal year							Total
	2002	2003	2004	2005	2006	2007	2008	
Inspections where problems were identified[b]	40	47	86	116	82	52	25	**448**
Total number of inspecttions	70	88	196	206	155	128	66	**909**
Percentage of inspections where investigators identifyied problems	57.1%	53.4%	43.9%	56.3%	52.9%	40.6%	37.9%	**49.3%**

Source: GAO analysis of FDA data.

[a] Dietary supplement inspections excludes those inspections related to dietary supplements with drug or veterinary uses.

[b] Problems identified includes both potential violations, as well as observations of problems by investigators that may fall below FDA's threshold for regulatory action.

Data on FDA's Actions to Respond to Safety Concerns Related to Dietary Supplements

FDA actions to respond to safety concerns related to dietary supplements include issuing warning letters to dietary supplement firms, requesting recalls, and detaining and refusing imports.

Data on Dietary Supplement-Related Warning Letters

Table 14 shows the number of Federal Food, Drug, and Cosmetic Act violations cited in 293 dietary supplement-related warning letters issued from fiscal years 2002 through 2007.

Table 15 shows the number of dietary supplement-related warning letters compared with total warning letters issued by FDA from fiscal years 2002 through 2007.

Table 14. Number of Violations in the Federal Food, Drug, and Cosmetic Act Cited in 293 FDA Dietary Supplement-Related Warning Letters, Fiscal Years 2002 through 2007

Violation description	Federal Food, Drug, and Cosmetic Act section	Number of violations in the 293 letters	Percentage of total violations
Unapproved new drug—product lacks FDA approval to manufacture and sell as a drug.	505	219	41.0%
Misbranded drug—product label is false or misleading, lacks adequate directions for use, or otherwise does not meet other drug labeling requirements.	502	153	28.7
Misbranded food—product label is false or misleading, bears unauthorized claims, does not list all ingredients, lacks required nutrition information, or does not meet other food labeling requirements.	403	136	25.5
Adulterated food—product contains ingredients that are unsafe, fraudulent, unapproved, or otherwise unfit for food.	402	9	1.7
Unapproved food additive—product contains a food additive that lacks FDA approval or that is not used in conformity with the regulation prescribing conditions for safe use of the additive.	409	4	0.7
Drug facility registration—firm failed to register its manufacturing facility with FDA as a drug facility.	510	4	0.7
Import or export violations—product violates import or export requirements.	801	3	0.6
Food contaminated with pesticides—product contains unsafe type or level of pesticides.	408	2	0.4
New dietary ingredient—product contains a new dietary ingredient that lacks adequate information to provide reasonable assurance of safety.	413	2	0.4
Food facility registration—firm failed to register as a food facility.	415	1	0.2
Prescription needed—firm failed to require dispensation of product by prescription.	503	1	0.2
Total violations		534	100.0%

Source: GAO analysis of FDA's online database of warning letters.

Note: Because FDA's online database may not include all the warning letters issued by FDA, these numbers represent minimums only.

Table 15. FDA Dietary Supplement-Related Warning Letters and All Other FDA Warning Letters Issued, Fiscal Years 2002 through 2007

Description	Fiscal year						Total
	2002	2003	2004	2005	2006	2007	
Dietary supplement letters	23	67	38	52	70	43	**293**
Total warning letters	806	761	730	519	526	434	**3,776**
Percentage of total warning letters	2.9%	8.8%	5.2%	10.0%	13.3%	9.9%	**7.8%**

Source: GAO analysis of FDA's online database of warning letters.

Note: Because FDA's online database may not include all the warning letters issued by FDA, these numbers represent minimums only. In addition to warning letters, FDA also sent untitled letters to dietary supplement companies for violations that did not meet the threshold of regulatory significance to trigger a warning letter. According to FDA, the agency sent approximately 240 untitled letters from 2003 through 2007.

Data on Recalls Related to Dietary Supplements

Table 16 provides information on examples of Class I recalls related to dietary supplement products from fiscal years 2003 through 2008. According to FDA, Class I recalls are related to products that are dangerous and defective and pose a serious health concern. A firm may initiate a recall independently of FDA, or FDA may request a firm recall a product upon identifying a problem with a product.

Table 16. Examples of Dietary Supplement-Related Class I Recalls, Fiscal Years 2003 through 2008

Fiscal year by recall date	Reason for recall	Product description
2003	Misbranded—product claims to be dairy-free when it contains a milk derivative.	Calcium / vitamin D supplement
2003	Unapproved new drug—product contains pharmaceutical for erectile dysfunction.	Supplements promoted for sexual function.
2003	Unapproved new drug—product contains pharmaceutical for erectile dysfunction.	Supplements promoted for sexual function.
2003	Unapproved new drug—product contains pharmaceutical for erectile dysfunction.	Herbal supplement promoted for sexual function.
2003	Unapproved new drug—product contains pharmaceutical for erectile dysfunction.	Herbal supplement promoted for sexual function.

Fiscal year by recall date	Reason for recall	Product description
2003	Unapproved new drug—product contains pharmaceutical for erectile dysfunction.	Herbal supplement promoted for sexual function.
2004	Misbranded—product contains excessive level of vitamin D.	Multivitamin
2005	Unapproved new drug—product contains pharmaceutical for erectile dysfunction.	Supplement promoted for sexual function.
2005	Adulterated—products contain aristolochic acid, a potent carcinogen and toxin.	Herbal supplements
2005	Unapproved new drug—product contains pharmaceutical for erectile dysfunction.	Supplement promoted for sexual function.
2005	Misbranded—product contains undeclared milk derivative.	Children's chewable calcium tablets
2005	Unapproved new drug—product prescripttion drug for treating Type 2 diabetes.	Herbal supplement
2005	Adulterated—product contains ephedrine alkaloids.	Supplement promoted for energy increase.
2006	Adulterated—product contains ephedrine alkaloids.	Supplement promoted for weight loss.
2006	Misbranded—product contains undeclared milk derivatives.	Calcium supplement
2006	Unapproved new drug—product contains analog of pharmaceutical for erectile dysfunction.	Herbal supplement promoted for sexual function.
2006	Unapproved new drug—product contains analog of pharmaceutical for erectile dysfunction.	Herbal supplement promoted for sexual function.
2007	Unapproved new drug—product contains analog of pharmaceutical for erectile dysfunction.	Herbal supplement promoted for sexual function.
2007	Unapproved new drug—product contains pharmaceutical for erectile dysfunction.	Supplement promoted for sexual function.
2007	Unapproved new drug—product contains analog of pharmaceutical for erectile dysfunction.	Herbal supplement promoted for sexual function.
2007	Misbranded—product may contain undeclared milk protein.	Protein supplement
2007	Misbranded—product contains undeclared milk.	Protein supplement
2007	Misbranded—product contains undeclared milk derivative.	Protein supplement
2007	Unapproved new drug—product contains analog of pharmaceutical for erectile dysfunction.	Supplement promoted for sexual function.
2007	Misbranded—product contains undeclared fish gelatin.	Multivitamin

Table 16. (Continued)

Fiscal year by recall date	Reason for recall	Product description
2007	Unapproved new drug—product contains analogs of various pharmaceuticals for erectile dysfunction.	Herbal supplement promoted for energy increase and male sexual function.
2007	Unapproved new drug—product contains analog of pharmaceutical for erectile dysfunction.	Herbal supplement promoted for sexual function.
2007	Adulterated—product may contain salmonella.	Shark cartilage supplement
2007	Adulterated—product may contain salmonella.	Shark cartilage supplement
2007	Misbranded—product contains undeclared soy.	Calcium supplement
2007	Unapproved new drug—product contains pharmaceutical for erectile dysfunction.	Supplement promoted for sexual function.
2007	Adulterated—product may contain salmonella.	Shark cartilage supplement
2007	Unapproved new drug—product contains pharmaceutical for weight loss.	Supplement promoted for weight loss.
2007	Unapproved new drug—product contains analogs of various pharmaceuticals for erectile dysfunction.	Supplements promoted for increasing sexual function.
2007	Unapproved new drug—product contains analogs of various pharmaceuticals for erectile dysfunction.	Supplements promoted for increasing sexual function.
2007	Adulterated—product contains cryptosporidium, a parasite that can cause intestinal infection, reported illness associated with product.	Herbal supplement promo-ted for treating upset stomach in infants.
2008	Adulterated—product may be contaminated with mold.	Folic acid liquid supplement
2008	Unapproved new drug—product contains analog of pharmaceutical for erectile dysfunction.	Supplement promoted for sexual function.
2008	Unapproved new drug—product contains analog of pharmaceutical for erectile dysfunction.	Supplement promoted for sexual function.
2008	Adulterated—product contains elevated levels of selenium and chromium, reported illnesses associated with the product.	Liquid dietary supplement
2008	Unapproved new drug—product contains various pharmaceuticals for erectile dysfunction.	Herbal supplement promoted for sexual function.
2008	Unapproved new drug—product contains analog of pharmaceutical for erectile dysfunction.	Supplement promoted for sexual function.
2008	Unapproved new drug—product contains analog of pharmaceutical for erectile	Herbal supplement promoted for sexual function.

Fiscal year by recall date	Reason for recall	Product description
	dysfunction.	
2008	Unapproved new drug—product contains pharmaceutical for erectile dysfunction.	Herbal supplement promoted for sexual function.
2008	Unapproved new drug—product contains analog of pharmaceutical for erectile dysfunction.	Herbal supplement promoted for sexual function.

Source: GAO analysis of FDA data available on FDA's Web site.

Note: These recalls are only examples of Class I recalls during this time period. We could not provide complete data on the number of recalls because FDA's official recalls database was not sufficiently reliable for the purposes of this report.

Table 17. Dietary Supplement-Related Detentions without Physical Examination (DWPE) by General Violation Categories, Fiscal Year 2002 through March 24, 2008[a]

Violation description	Dietary supplement entry lines DWPE	Percentage of total violations for dietary supplement import entry lines DWPE
Adulterated—product appears to contain an unsafe substance, or appears to have been prepared under insanitary conditions or in a facility that lacks manufacturing controls or does not otherwise meet FDA regulations.	1,623	50.3%
Misbranded—product label appears to be false or misleading, or appears to not meet labeling requirements.	1,109	34.4
Unapproved new drug—product appears to lack FDA approval to manufacture and sell as a drug.	324	10.0
Other	162	5.0
Adulterated—firm appears to have unlawfully omitted or substituted an ingredient in the product.	7	0.2
Total	**3,225**	**100.0%**

Source: GAO analysis of FDA data.

[a] When identifiable, this table excludes products for animal uses, topical products, cosmetics, and other products that do not meet the statutory definition of a dietary supplement. Data includes dietary supplement products for drug uses.

Data on Imports Related to Dietary Supplements

Table 17 shows the number of detentions without physical examination of imported dietary supplement products by general violation categories from fiscal year 2002 through March 24, 2008.

Table 18 shows the number of detentions without physical examination of imported dietary supplement products by product classification from fiscal year 2002 through March 24, 2008.

Table 18. Dietary Supplement-Related DWPE by Product Classification, Fiscal Year 2002 through March 24, 2008[a]

Product classification[b]	Dietary supplement entry lines DWPE	Percentage of dietary supplement entry lines DWPE
Herbal and botanical (other than teas)	1,049	32.5%
Herbal and botanical teas	750	23.3
Vitamin	628	19.5
Protein	527	16.3
Animal by-products and extracts	136	4.2
Combination products and products not elsewhere classified	54	1.7
Mineral	36	1.1
Other	25	0.8
Fats and lipid substances	20	0.6
Total	**3,225**	**100.0%**

Source: GAO analysis of FDA data.

[a] When identifiable, this table excludes products for animal uses, topical products, cosmetics, and other products that do not meet the statutory definition of a dietary supplement. Data includes dietary supplement products for drug uses.

[b] Product classifications for import entry lines are submitted by customs brokers and are not determined by FDA unless reviewed and corrected during an examination. Accordingly, some entry lines may be incorrectly classified.

Table 19 shows the number of Federal Food, Drug, and Cosmetic Act violations cited in 3,605 dietary supplement-related import refusals from fiscal year 2002 through March 24, 2008.

Table 19. Number of Violations of the Federal Food, Drug, and Cosmetic Act Cited in 3,605 Dietary Supplement-Related Import Refusals, Fiscal Year 2002 through March 24, 2008[a]

Violation description	Number of violations for the 3,605 lines refused	Percentage of total violations
Misbranded—product label appears to be false or misleading, or appears to not meet labeling requirements.	3,193	57.4%
Adulterated—product appears to contain an unsafe substance, or appears to have been prepared under insanitary conditions or in a facility that lacks manufacturing controls or does not otherwise meet FDA regulations.	1,366	24.6
Unapproved new drug—product appears to lack FDA approval to manufacture and sell as a drug.	730	13.1
Other	258	4.6
Adulterated—firm appears to have unlawfully omitted or substituted an ingredient in the product.	13	0.2
Total	**5,560**	**100.0%**

Source: GAO analysis of FDA data.

[a] When identifiable, this table excludes products for animal uses, topical products, cosmetics, and other products that do not meet the statutory definition of a dietary supplement. Data includes dietary supplement products for drug uses.

Table 20 shows the number of refused imports of dietary supplement products by product classification from fiscal year 2002 through March 24, 2008.

Table 20. Dietary Supplement-Related Import Refusals by Product Classification, Fiscal Year 2002 through March 24, 2008[a]

Product classification[b]	Dietary supplement entry lines refused	Percentage of dietary supplement entry lines refused
Herbal and botanical (other than teas)	1,378	38.2%
Combination products, and products not elsewhere classified	900	25.0
Herbal and botanical teas	569	15.8
Vitamin	408	11.3
Animal by-products and extracts	111	3.1
Protein	71	2.0

Table 20. (Continued)

Product classification[b]	Dietary supplement entry lines refused	Percentage of dietary supplement entry lines refused
Mineral	65	1.8
Other	59	1.6
Fats and lipid substances	43	1.2
Total	**3,604**	**100.0%**

Source: GAO analysis of FDA data.

[a] When identifiable, this table excludes products for animal uses, topical products, cosmetics, and other products that do not meet the statutory definition of a dietary supplement. Data includes dietary supplement products for drug uses.

[b] Product classifications for import entry lines are submitted by customs brokers and are not determined by FDA unless reviewed and corrected during an examination. Accordingly, some entry lines may be incorrectly classified.

Data on FDA Enforcement Actions Related to Dietary Supplements

FDA's enforcement actions related to dietary supplements include seizures, injunctions, and criminal investigations. Table 21 shows information about dietary supplement-related seizure and injunction actions taken from fiscal year 2002 through July 18, 2008.

Table 22 summarizes dietary supplement-related criminal investigations resulting in at least one conviction or with charges filed from 2002 through July 31, 2008.

Table 21. FDA Seizures and Injunctions Related to Dietary Supplement Products, Fiscal Year 2002 through July 18, 2008[a]

Fiscal year	Type of action	Date filed	Individual/company	Product description	Reason	Note
2002	Seizure	10/22/2001	Biogenics Inc.; E'OLA International; and Nature's Energy, Inc.	Various weight-loss products	Unapproved new drug/misbranded drug	
2002	Seizure	2/5/2002	Spectramin, Inc.	Various products for joint health, vitality, energy, and weight loss, among others	Unapproved new drug/misbranded drug	
2002	Seizure	6/10/2002	Dandy Day Corporation	Product promoted for weight loss.	Unapproved new drug/misbranded drug	
2002	Seizure	9/25/2002	Zibo Fuxing PharmacyCo, Ltd./Sino King International Development and Management Group, Inc.	Herbal product to treat or prevent me-ntal development disorders and diseases.	Misbranded food, unapproved new drug/Misbr-anded drug	
2003	Seizure	10/15/2002	Humphrey Laboratories, Inc., Kirkman Laboratories	Product to treat or prevent autism.	Misbranded food, unapproved new drug/-misbranded drug	
2003	Seizure	12/13/2002	Halo Supply, Co.	Product to treat or prevent cold, flu, and other viral conditions.	Unapproved new drug/misbranded drug	
2003	Seizure	2/4/2003	Global Source Management and Consulting Inc.	Various products promoted to treat or prevent medical conditions, including enlarged prostate, joint health, and chole-sterol reduction.	Unapproved new drug/misbranded drug	

Table 21. (Continued)

Fiscal year	Type of action	Date filed	Individual/company	Product description	Reason	Note
2003	Seizure	6/16/2003	Seasilver USA, Inc. (Southern District of California)	Product promoted to treat or prevent hypoglycemia, diabetes, cancer, psoriasis, hepatictis, and arthritis.	Misbranded food, unapproved new drug/Misbranded drug	Related consent decree of condemnation and permanent injunction filed 3/9/04. Product was also seized from Ohio on 6/24/03.
2003	Seizure	6/19/2003	Shop America	Product promoted to treat or prevent cancer, heart disease, and various degenerative diseases.	Misbranded food, unapproved new drug/misbranded drug	Related consent decree of condemnation and permanent injunction filed 12/17/03.
2003	Injunction	9/16/2003	Hi-Tech Pharmaceuticals, National Urological Group, National Institute for Clinical Weight Loss, Americ-an Weight Loss Clinic, United Metabolic Research Center, and Jared R. Wheat	Various products promoted to treat or prevent obesity and erectile dysfunction.	Unapproved new drug/misbranded drug	
2003	Seizure	9/18/2003	Jean's Greens	Herbal product promoted to treat or prevent serious diseases, such as cancer.	Unapproved new drug/misbranded drug	
2004	Seizure	1/22/2004	EAS / Musclemaster.com, Inc., NVE Pharmaceuticals, Inc.	Various products promoted to build muscle mass.	Misbranded food	
2005	Seizure	11/22/2004	Asia MedLabs, Inc.	Herbal product to treat or prevent flu, poisoning, allergies, blood pressure, and other heart ailments.	Adulterated food, unapproved new drug/ misbranded drug	

Table 21. (Continued)

Fiscal year	Type of action	Date filed	Individual/company	Product description	Reason	Note
2005	Seizure	12/15/2004	FCC Products, Inc.	Ginseng contamina-ted with pesticides	Adulterated food	
2005	Seizure	2/11/2005	ATF Fitness Products, Inc.	Weight-loss products containing ephedra.	Adulterated food and misbranded food	
2006	Injunction	10/14/2005	Vita-ERB, Ltd. Mary and Moses Barnes and Fred Paulicka	Herbal product mar-keted with disease claims.	Unapproved new drug/misbranded drug, adulterated drug	
2006	Seizure	11/28/2005	Nature's Treat, Inc.	Product containing ephedra promoted for increasing energy.	Adulterated food	Products also seized at distributor on the same date.
2006	Seizure	1/9/2006	ATF Fitness Products, Inc.	Product containing ephedra.	Adulterated food	
2006	Injunction	2/3/2006	Natural Ovens Bakery, Paul and Barbara Stitt, Matthew Taylor	Various supplement mixes	Misbranded food, unapproved new drug/misbranded drug	Injunction included food products as well.
2006	Seizure	2/22/2006	Hi-Tech Pharmaceuticals, Inc.	Products contain-ing ephedra.	Adulterated food	
2006	Seizure	9/5/2006	Advantage Nutraceuticals, LLC	Various products including those promoted to treat or prevent cancer and arthritis.	Unapproved new drug/misbranded drug	

Table 21. (Continued)

Fiscal year	Type of action	Date filed	Individual/company	Product description	Reason	Note
2007	Seizure	12/29/2006	Vitality Products Co., Inc.	Various products promoted to treat or prevent serious diseases, such as cancer, heart disease, Alzheim-er's disease, and others.	Unapproved new drug/misbranded drug	
2007	Seizure	8/22/2007	Charron Nutrition	Various products promoted to treat or prevent diabetes, arthritis, and other serious medical conditions.	Unapproved new drug/misbranded drug	
2008	Seizure	10/18/2007	FulLife Natural Options, Inc.	Various products promoted to treat or prevent diabetes, anemia, and hyper-tension, among other conditions.	Unapproved new drug/misbranded drug	
2008	Seizure	10/29/2007	General Therapeutics, Corporation	Products manufact-ured under insane-itary conditions.	Unapproved new drug, adulterated drug, adulterated food	
2008	Injunction	2/12/2008	Brownwood Acres Foods Inc., Cherry Capital Servi-ces, Inc., Stephen de Tar, Robert Underwood	Various products promoted to treat or prevent cancer, arthritis, gout, heart disease, and Alzh-eimer's disease, among others.	Unapproved new drug/ misbranded drug, misbranded food	

Table 21. (Continued)

Fiscal year	Type of action	Date filed	Individual/company	Product description	Reason	Note
2008	Seizure	3/25/2008	Shangai Distributor, Inc.	Various products promoted for sexual enhancement and to treat erectile dysfunction.	Unapproved new drug/ misbranded drug	
2008	Seizure	4/2/2008	LG Sciences, LLC	Products promoted for bodybuilding and containing unapproved dietary ingredients and unapproved food additives.	Adulterated food	
2008	Seizure	7/18/2008	Sei Pharmaceuticals, Inc.	Various products promoted for sexual enhancement and to treat erectile dysfunction.	Unapproved new drug/misbranded drug	

Source: GAO analysis of FDA data.

[a] In some cases, FDA may have initiated multiple actions for a particular product such as seizing the same product from different companies or locations (e.g., distributor). These related actions are listed in the notes column.

Table 22. Number of Criminal Investigations Related to Dietary Supplements Resulting in a Conviction or Charges Filed from 2002 through July 31, 2008

Description	Number of cases
Cases resulting in at least one conviction (state or federal)	14
Cases with charges filed (state or federal)	5
Total	**19**

Source: GAO analysis of FDA data.

Note: Cases with charges filed includes cases where specific charges have been filed within the judicial system and indictments. This category excludes cases where charges may have been filed but the case was not pursued further (e.g., prosecution declined or case dismissed).

APPENDIX III: COMPARISON OF SELECT FOREIGN COUNTRIES' REGULATION OF DIETARY SUPPLEMENTS WITH THE UNITED STATES

In comparison with the United States, Canada and Japan have more regulatory requirements in place for dietary supplements and related products. On the other hand, the United States has developed specific good manufacturing practices for dietary supplements while the United Kingdom has not. Table 23 compares the regulatory framework for dietary supplement products in these foreign countries with the U.S. regulatory system.

Table 23. Comparison of Dietary Supplement Regulations: United States, Canada, United Kingdom, and Japan

Country	Product registration	Manufacturer registration	Premarket approval of products	Specific good manufacturing practices	Serious mandatory adverse event reporting by industry
United States		X (limited)		X	X
Canada	X	X[a]	X	X	X
United Kingdom		X	X[b] (limited)		X[c]
Japan[d]	X	X	X	X[e]	

Source: GAO.

Note: GAO did not independently verify descriptions of foreign laws.

[a] Manufacturers, packagers, labelers, and importers of natural health products must obtain a site license to perform these activities.

[b] Under European Community (E.C.) law, novel supplements without a history of consumption in the European Union prior to May 1997, or foods containing genetically-modified ingredients are subject to premarket approval for safety.

[c] According to a U.K. official, under E.C. law, firms must report any problems with products to the local and national authorities.

[d] Foods for Specified Health Uses (FOSHU) products only.

[e] According to a Japanese official, Japan does not have separate good manufacturing practice regulations for dietary supplement products; however, firms applying to use a FOSHU claim on a product must provide evidence that quality control procedures are in place for that particular product.

In Canada, companies are required to obtain a product license to market natural health products, which include a range of products, such as vitamin and mineral supplements, herbal remedies, and other products, based upon their medicinal ingredients and intended uses. The product licensing application must include detailed information about the product, ingredients, potency, intended use, and evidence supporting the product's safety and efficacy. Approved products are assigned a license number that is displayed on the product label. Manufacturers, packagers, labelers, and importers of natural health products must obtain a site license to perform these activities. To obtain a site license, a firm must provide evidence of quality control procedures that meet government standards for good manufacturing practices. Firms are required to report any serious adverse reactions associated with their products within 15 days and must provide information summarizing all adverse reactions, including mild or moderate events, on an annual basis.

In the United Kingdom (U.K.), dietary supplements are legally termed "food supplements" and are regulated under food law—most of which is European Community (E.C.) legislation implemented at the national level, according to a U.K. official. Food supplements are generally not subject to premarket approval. For example, any supplement that either meets the guidelines established under E.U. law for specific vitamins and minerals, or does not include a new or genetically modified ingredient, does not require approval prior to marketing. According to a U.K. official, most direct oversight of the dietary supplement industry in the United Kingdom occurs at the local level of government. For example, all investigations, enforcement actions, and monitoring activities such as inspections are undertaken at the local level. Food supplement firms are required to register with local authorities and should detail the specific activities undertaken at each establishment as part of this process. However, centralized information on registered firms is not collected or maintained at a national level. Additionally, there is no centralized registry of food supplement products in the U.K. Although government standards for food good manufacturing practices apply to food supplement manufacturing, there are no good manufacturing practice guidelines specific for food supplements. Under E.C. law, firms are required to report any problems with food products to the local and national authorities and, if the product is injurious to health, the firm must remove it from the market.

In Japan, products are regulated based on their product claims. There are two types of claims: Food with Nutrient Function Claims (FNFC), which are standardized, preapproved claim statements for certain vitamins and minerals with established benefits, and Food for Specified Health Uses (FOSHU) claims, which require government approval for safety and efficacy prior to marketing a product advertised as having a physiological effect on the body. Since FNFC claims are standardized and preapproved, firms do not need to notify the government prior to marketing a product using an approved FNFC claim, provided the product meets established ingredient content specifications. To use a FOSHU claim on a product, a firm is required to provide the government with evidence supporting the product's physiological effect and safety prior to marketing. Additionally, a firm must provide information on the firm and its product to the government, as well as evidence of quality control processes.

ppendix IV: Comments from the Department of Health and Human Services

DEPARTMENT OF HEALTH & HUMAN SERVICES   OFFICE OF THE SECRETARY

Assistant Secretary for Legislation
Washington, DC 20201

JAN 2 2 2009

Lisa Shames
Director, Natural Resources and Environment
U.S. Government Accountability Office
441 G Street N.W.
Washington, DC 20548

Dear Ms. Shames:

Enclosed are comments on the U.S. Government Accountability Office's (GAO) report entitled:
"Dietary Supplements:FDA Should Take Further Actions to Improve Oversight and Consumer
Understanding, (GAO-09-250).

The Department appreciates the opportunity to review this report before its publication.

Sincerely,

Barbara Pisaro Clark

Barbara Pisaro Clark
Acting Assistant Secretary for Legislation

Attachment

DEPARTMENT OF HEALTH & HUMAN SERVICES

Food and Drug Administration
Silver Spring, MD 20993

January 22, 2009

To: Assistant Secretary for Legislation

From: FDA Chief of Staff

Subject: FDA's General Comments to the U.S. Government Accountability
Office's (GAO) Draft Report Entitled: *Dietary Supplements: FDA
Should Take Further Actions to Improve Oversight and Consumer
Understanding* (GAO-09-250)

FDA is providing the attached general comments to the U.S. Government Accountability
Office's draft report entitled, *Dietary Supplements: FDA Should Take Further Actions to
Improve Oversight and Consumer Understanding (GAO-09-250)*.

We appreciate the opportunity to review and comment on this draft correspondence
before it is published.

Susan C. Winckler, R.Ph., Esq.

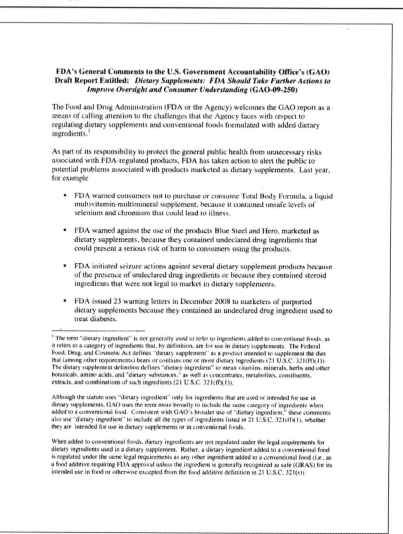

FDA's General Comments to the U.S. Government Accountability Office's (GAO) Draft Report Entitled: *Dietary Supplements: FDA Should Take Further Actions to Improve Oversight and Consumer Understanding* **(GAO-09-250)**

The Food and Drug Administration (FDA or the Agency) welcomes the GAO report as a means of calling attention to the challenges that the Agency faces with respect to regulating dietary supplements and conventional foods formulated with added dietary ingredients.[1]

As part of its responsibility to protect the general public health from unnecessary risks associated with FDA-regulated products, FDA has taken action to alert the public to potential problems associated with products marketed as dietary supplements. Last year, for example

- FDA warned consumers not to purchase or consume Total Body Formula, a liquid multivitamin-multimineral supplement, because it contained unsafe levels of selenium and chromium that could lead to illness.

- FDA warned against the use of the products Blue Steel and Hero, marketed as dietary supplements, because they contained undeclared drug ingredients that could present a serious risk of harm to consumers using the products.

- FDA initiated seizure actions against several dietary supplement products because of the presence of undeclared drug ingredients or because they contained steroid ingredients that were not legal to market in dietary supplements.

- FDA issued 23 warning letters in December 2008 to marketers of purported dietary supplements because they contained an undeclared drug ingredient used to treat diabetes.

---

[1] The term "dietary ingredient" is not generally used to refer to ingredients added to conventional foods, as it refers to a category of ingredients that, by definition, are for use in dietary supplements. The Federal Food, Drug, and Cosmetic Act defines "dietary supplement" as a product intended to supplement the diet that (among other requirements) bears or contains one or more dietary ingredients (21 U.S.C. 321(ff)(1)). The dietary supplement definition defines "dietary ingredient" to mean vitamins, minerals, herbs and other botanicals, amino acids, and "dietary substances," as well as concentrates, metabolites, constituents, extracts, and combinations of such ingredients (21 U.S.C. 321(ff)(1)).

Although the statute uses "dietary ingredient" only for ingredients that are used or intended for use in dietary supplements, GAO uses the term more broadly to include the same category of ingredients when added to a conventional food. Consistent with GAO's broader use of "dietary ingredient," these comments also use "dietary ingredient" to include all the types of ingredients listed in 21 U.S.C. 321(ff)(1), whether they are intended for use in dietary supplements or in conventional foods.

When added to conventional foods, dietary ingredients are not regulated under the legal requirements for dietary ingredients used in a dietary supplement. Rather, a dietary ingredient added to a conventional food is regulated under the same legal requirements as any other ingredient added to a conventional food (i.e., as a food additive requiring FDA approval unless the ingredient is generally recognized as safe (GRAS) for its intended use in food or otherwise excepted from the food additive definition in 21 U.S.C. 321(s)).

- FDA continued to identify and take enforcement action against dietary supplements making illegal disease treatment claims. For example, between June and September 2008 FDA issued 28 warning letters to firms that were marketing fake cancer cures, many of which were marketed as dietary supplements.

- FDA continues to make progress toward accomplishing other related tasks, even though funding is limited. As noted in the current draft report, FDA issued draft guidance to implement the labeling, reporting, and recordkeeping provisions of the Dietary Supplement and Nonprescription Drug Consumer Protection Act, and FDA took steps to update internal systems and processes for collecting and analyzing serious adverse event reports submitted to FDA.

GAO Recommendation 1

To improve the information available to FDA for identifying safety concerns and better enable FDA to meet its responsibility to protect the public health, we recommend that the Secretary of the Department of Health and Human Services direct the Commissioner of FDA to request authority to require dietary supplement companies to

- Identify themselves as a dietary supplement company as part of the existing registration requirements and update this information annually.
- Provide a list of all dietary supplement products they sell and a copy of the labels and update this information annually, and
- Report all adverse events related to dietary supplements.

FDA Response to Recommendation 1

In general, FDA agrees that the Agency's ability to ensure the safety of dietary supplements used by consumers could be improved if FDA had more information on the identity of firms marketing dietary supplements as well as the identity and composition of the products they market. However, it is not clear that all the information would actually enhance product safety. For example, the GAO draft report recommends that FDA require firms to report *all* adverse events related to dietary supplements. Although receiving all adverse events on dietary supplements could theoretically enhance our ability to detect signals of potential toxicity over time, we are uncertain whether, in practice, such information would advance the Agency's ability to identify unsafe dietary supplements or to do so quickly. For example, an unintended outcome of receiving such reports might be that the huge increase in minor adverse event reports might make it more difficult to filter out signals of potential toxicity generated by reports of serious adverse events and thus delay the identification of safety problems with dietary supplements. However, FDA is working on methodologies to try to mitigate this concern and improve data mining for safety-related signals if the Agency were to receive *all* adverse event reports.

2

GAO Recommendation 2

To better enable FDA to meet its responsibility to regulate dietary supplements that contain new dietary ingredients, we recommend that the Secretary of the Department of Health and Human Services direct the Commissioner of FDA to issue guidance to clarify when an ingredient is considered a new dietary ingredient, the evidence needed to document the safety of new dietary ingredients, and appropriate methods for establishing ingredient identity.

FDA Response to Recommendation 2

FDA agrees that guidance would be helpful to clarify when an ingredient is considered a new dietary ingredient (NDI), the evidence needed to document the safety of NDIs, and appropriate methods for establishing the identity of a NDI. The Agency held a public meeting in November 2004 to seek public comment on several issues related to the NDI requirements of section 413(a)(2) of the Federal Food, Drug, and Cosmetic Act (21 U.S.C. 350b(a)(2)). FDA specifically asked for information that would enable the Agency to identify ways to assist submitters of NDI notifications to ensure that they contain the information the Agency needs to evaluate the notification and to clarify statutory requirements in the Dietary Supplement Health and Education Act of 1994 (DSHEA) that pertain to NDIs. The Agency has reviewed the information submitted by interested parties on this subject and has developed draft guidance addressing the NDI notification requirements of the Federal Food, Drug, and Cosmetic Act. The guidance is currently undergoing internal FDA review.

GAO Recommendation 3

To help ensure that companies follow the appropriate laws and regulations and renew a recommendation we made in July 2000, we recommend that the Secretary of the Department of Health and Human Services direct the Commissioner of FDA to provide guidance to industry to clarify when products should be marketed as either dietary supplements or foods with added dietary ingredients.

FDA Response to Recommendation 3

As we noted in our comment to the GAO July 2000 report, FDA's Dietary Supplement Strategic Plan recognized the need to clarify the boundaries between dietary supplements and conventional foods, including conventional foods with added dietary ingredients. As we noted when the Plan was released in January 2000, FDA acknowledged its inability to set timeframes for all the activities listed in the Plan because of resource limitations. FDA will consider this recommendation and the priority and timing to implement this recommendation in light of the Agency's limited resources and competing priorities.

3

GAO Recommendation 4

To improve consumer understanding about dietary supplements and better leverage existing resources, we recommend that the Secretary of the Department of Health and Human Services direct the Commissioner of FDA to coordinate with stakeholder groups involved in consumer outreach to (1) identify additional mechanisms—such as the recent WebMD partnership—for educating consumers about the safety, efficacy, and labeling of dietary supplements, (2) implement these mechanisms, and (3) assess their effectiveness.

FDA Response to Recommendation 4

In principle, FDA agrees that more information about the use of dietary supplements would help consumers who are trying to determine whether the use of a particular supplement is safe or desirable in light of their personal health. However, the Agency is unsure that FDA is best situated to meet this consumer need. Although FDA does, as the report notes, engage in some consumer education and outreach, our resources available for this type of activity are extremely limited. Moreover, DSHEA recognized that the National Institutes of Health (NIH) is well situated to undertake the resource-intensive task of conducting and compiling scientific research on dietary supplements, dietary ingredients, and their effects on the body. In fact, the NIH's Office of Dietary Supplements offers a number of consumer-oriented Fact Sheets, databases of dietary supplement research activities, and literature citations, for the purpose of educating the public to foster an enhanced quality of life and health for the U.S. population. Thus, FDA believes that it may be useful to explore a possible collaboration between FDA and NIH as an efficient and cost-effective way to expand and further our current outreach activities on dietary supplements. FDA also believes that collaboration with other stakeholders may be useful for communicating information on the safety and uses of dietary supplements to the general public. In this regard, FDA is identifying areas of consumer information appropriate for the recently announced FDA/WebMD partnership, referenced in the GAO report. We anticipate that information on dietary supplements will be included.

4

r/d: ONLDS, BMoore, BFrankos: 1/5/09
Clearance ONLDS, MPoos:1/5/09
Edits: NYanish: 1/6/09
Edits: HSeltzer: 1/6/09
Edits: DCooper: 1/6/09
Edits: TMattia: 1/6/09
Edits: ACrawford: 1/6/09
Edits & Review: ONLDS, BMoore, BFrankos, MPoos: 1/7/09
Edits & EOS Clearance: BHarden, 1/7/09
Edit: MPoos/BFrankos, 1/8/09
Edits/Clearance: MLanda, 1/9/09
Edits/CGrillo 1/14/09
Edited LNickerson 1/15/09
Reviewed CGrillo 1/16/09
Edits and OFP Clearance CNelson 1/21/09
Edited D.Foellmer 1/21/09
Edited P. Quest at NIH 1/22/09

5

APPENDIX V: GAO CONTACT AND STAFF ACKNOWLEDGMENTS

GAO Contact

Lisa Shames, (202) 512-3841, shamesl@gao.gov

Staff Acknowledgments

In addition to the individual named above, José Alfredo Gómez, Assistant Director; Kevin Bray; Nancy Crothers; Michele Fejfar; Alison Gerry Grantham; Barbara Patterson; Minette Richardson; Lisa Van Arsdale; and Chloe Wardropper made key contributions to this report.

GAO'S MISSION

The Government Accountability Office, the audit, evaluation, and investigative arm of Congress, exists to support Congress in meeting its constitutional responsibilities and to help improve the performance and accountability of the federal government for the American people. GAO examines the use of public funds; evaluates federal programs and policies; and provides analyses, recommendations, and other assistance to help Congress make informed oversight, policy, and funding decisions. GAO's commitment to good government is reflected in its core values of accountability, integrity, and reliability.

OBTAINING COPIES OF GAO REPORTS AND TESTIMONY

The fastest and easiest way to obtain copies of GAO documents at no cost is through GAO's Web site (www.gao.gov). Each weekday afternoon, GAO posts on its Web site newly released reports, testimony, and correspondence. To have GAO e-mail you a list of newly posted products, go to www.gao.gov and select "E-mail Updates."

Order by Phone

The price of each GAO publication reflects GAO's actual cost of production and distribution and depends on the number of pages in the publication and whether the publication is printed in color or black and white. Pricing and ordering information is posted on GAO's Web site, http://www.gao.gov/ordering.htm.

Place orders by calling (202) 512-6000, toll free (866) 801-7077, or TDD (202) 512-2537.

Orders may be paid for using American Express, Discover Card, MasterCard, Visa, check, or money order. Call for additional information.

TO REPORT FRAUD, WASTE, AND ABUSE IN FEDERAL PROGRAMS

Contact: Web site: www.gao.gov/fraudnet/fraudnet.htm
E-mail: fraudnet@gao.gov
Automated answering system: (800) 424-5454 or (202) 512-7470

CONGRESSIONAL RELATIONS

Ralph Dawn, Managing Director, dawnr@gao.gov, (202) 512-4400 U.S. Government Accountability Office, 441 G Street NW, Room 7125 Washington, DC 20548

PUBLIC AFFAIRS

Chuck Young, Managing Director, youngc1@gao.gov, (202) 512-4800 U.S. Government Accountability Office, 441 G Street NW, Room 7149 Washington, DC 20548

End Notes

[1] GAO, *Food Safety: Improvements Needed in Overseeing the Safety of Dietary Supplements and "Functional Foods,"* GAO/RCED-00-156 (Washington, D.C.: July 11, 2000).

[2] Department of Health and Human Services Office of Inspector General, *Dietary Supplement Labels: An Assessment* (Washington, D.C.: March 2003).

[3] FDA's estimate was published in the *Federal Register* on September 15, 2008, in accordance with the Paperwork Reduction Act of 1995. The estimate is based on a 2000 FDA-commissioned study that examined factors affecting adverse event reporting for drugs and vaccines and then qualitatively assessed the potential impact of those factors for voluntary dietary supplement adverse event reporting.

[4] For more information on food inspections performed under state contract agreements, see GAO, *Food Labeling: FDA Needs to Better Leverage Resources, Improve Oversight, and Effectively Use Available Data to Help Consumers Select Healthy Foods*, GAO-08-597 (Washington, D.C.: Sept. 9, 2008).

[5] Department of Health and Human Services, U.S. Food and Drug Administration, Food Protection Plan: *An Integrated Strategy for Protecting the Nation's Food Supply* (Washington, D.C.: November 2007).

[6] Reports of mild or moderate reactions to dietary supplements may be considered a serious adverse event report if, based on reasonable medical judgment, a medical intervention was necessary to prevent a serious outcome.

[7] For more information on FDA resources by Center, see GAO, *Food Safety: Improvements Needed in FDA Oversight of Fresh Produce*, GAO-08-1047 (Washington, D.C.: Sept. 26, 2008).

[8] For more information on foreign inspections conducted by FDA, see GAO, *Federal Oversight of Food Safety: FDA Has Provided Few Details on the Resources and Strategies Needed to Implement its Food Protection Plan*, GAO-08-909T (Washington, D.C.: June 12, 2008).

[9] Department of Health and Human Services' Office of Inspector General, *Dietary Supplement Labels: An Assessment* (Washington, D.C.: March 2003).

In: Dietary Supplements: Primer and FDA...   ISBN: 978-1-60741-891-7
Editors: Timothy H. Riley   © 2010 Nova Science Publishers, Inc.

Chapter 3

FDA 101: DIETARY SUPPLEMENTS

U.S. Food and Drug Administration

The law defines dietary supplements in part as products taken by mouth that contain a "dietary ingredient." Dietary ingredients include vitamins, minerals, amino acids, and herbs or botanicals, as well as other substances that can be used to supplement the diet.

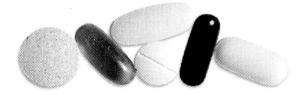

Dietary supplements come in many forms, including tablets, capsules, powders, energy bars, and liquids. These products are available in stores throughout the United States, as well as on the Internet. They are labeled as dietary supplements and include among others

- vitamin and mineral products
- "botanical" or herbal products—These come in many forms and may include plant materials, algae, macroscopic fungi, or a combination of these materials.

- amino acid products—Amino acids are known as the building blocks of proteins and play a role in metabolism.
- enzyme supplements—Enzymes are complex proteins that speed up biochemical reactions.

People use dietary supplements for a wide assortment of reasons. Some seek to compensate for diets, medical conditions, or eating habits that limit the intake of essential vitamins and nutrients. Other people look to them to boost energy or to get a good night's sleep. Postmenopausal women consider using them to counter a sudden drop in estrogen levels.

Talk with a Health Care Professional

The Food and Drug Administration (FDA) suggests that you consult with a health care professional before using any dietary supplement. Many supplements contain ingredients that have strong biological effects, and such products may not be safe in all people.

FDA suggests that you consult with a health care professional before using any dietary supplement. Using supplements improperly can be harmful. Taking a combination of supplements, using these products together with medicine, or substituting them in place of prescribed medicines could lead to harmful, even life-threatening, results.

If you have certain health conditions and take these products, you may be putting yourself at risk. Your health care professional can discuss with you whether it is safe for you to take a particular product and whether the product is appropriate for your needs. Here is some general advice:

- **Dietary supplements are not intended to treat, diagnose, cure, or alleviate the effects of diseases.** They cannot completely prevent diseases, as some vaccines can. However, some supplements are useful in reducing the risk of certain diseases and are authorized to make label claims about these uses. For example, folic acid supplements may make a claim about reducing the risk of birth defects of the brain and spinal cord.

- **Using supplements improperly can be harmful.** Taking a combination of supplements, using these products together with medicine, or substituting them in place of prescribed medicines could lead to harmful, even life-threatening, results.

- **Some supplements can have unwanted effects before, during, or after surgery.** For example, bleeding is a potential side effect risk of garlic, ginkgo biloba, ginseng, and Vitamin E. In addition, kava and valerian act as sedatives and can increase the effects of anesthetics and other medications used during surgery. Before surgery, you should inform your health care professional about all the supplements you use.

How Are Supplements Regulated?

You should know the following if you are considering using a dietary supplement.

- Federal law requires that every dietary supplement be labeled as such, either with the term "dietary supplement" or with a term that substitutes a description of the product's dietary ingredient(s) for the word "dietary" (e.g., "herbal supplement" or "calcium supplement").
- Federal law does not require dietary supplements to be proven safe to FDA's satisfaction before they are marketed.
- For most claims made in the labeling of dietary supplements, the law does not require the manufacturer or seller to prove to FDA's satisfaction that the claim is accurate or truthful before it appears on the product.
- In general, FDA's role with a dietary supplement product begins after the product enters the marketplace. That is usually the agency's first opportunity to take action against a product that presents a significant or unreasonable risk of illness or injury, or that is otherwise adulterated or misbranded.
- Dietary supplement advertising, including ads broadcast on radio and television, falls under the jurisdiction of the Federal Trade Commission.

- Once a dietary supplement is on the market, FDA has certain safety monitoring responsibilities. These include monitoring mandatory reporting of serious adverse events by dietary supplement firms and voluntary adverse event reporting by consumers and health care professionals. As its resources permit, FDA also reviews product labels and other product information, such as package inserts, accompanying literature, and Internet promotion.
- Dietary supplement firms must report to FDA any serious adverse events that are reported to them by consumers or health care professionals.
- Dietary supplement manufacturers do not have to get the agency's approval before producing or selling these products.
- It is not legal to market a dietary supplement product as a treatment or cure for a specific disease, or to alleviate the symptoms of a disease.
- There are limitations to FDA oversight of claims in dietary supplement labeling. For example, FDA reviews substantiation for claims as resources permit.

Are Supplements Safe?

Many dietary supplements have clean safety histories. For example, millions of Americans responsibly consume multi-vitamins and experience no ill effects.

Some dietary supplements have been shown to be beneficial for certain health conditions. For example, the use of folic acid supplements by women of childbearing age who may become pregnant reduces the risk of some birth defects.

Another example is the crystalline form of vitamin B12, which is beneficial in people over age 50 who often have a reduced ability to absorb naturally occurring vitamin B12. But further study is needed for some other dietary supplements.

Some ingredients and products can be harmful when consumed in high amounts, when taken for a long time, or when used in combination with certain other drugs, substances, or foods.

Some supplements have had to be recalled because of proven or potential harmful effects. Reasons for these recalls include

- microbiological, pesticide, and heavy metal contamination
- absence of a dietary ingredient claimed to be in the product
- the presence of more or less than the amount of the dietary ingredient claimed on the label

In addition, unscrupulous manufacturers have tried to sell bogus products that should not be on the market at all.

Before taking a dietary supplement, make sure that the supplement is safe for you and appropriate for the intended purpose.

Be a Safe and Informed Consumer

- Let your health care professional advise you on sorting reliable information from questionable information.
- Contact the manufacturer for information about the product you intend to use.
- Be aware that some supplement ingredients, including nutrients and plant components, can be toxic. Also, some ingredients and products can be harmful when consumed in high amounts, when taken for a long time, or when used in combination with certain other drugs, substances, or foods.
- Do not self-diagnose any health condition. Work with health care professionals to determine how best to achieve optimal health.
- Do not substitute a dietary supplement for a prescription medicine or therapy, or for the variety of foods important to a healthful diet.
- Do not assume that the term "natural" in relation to a product ensures that the product is wholesome or safe.
- Be wary of hype and headlines. Sound health advice is generally based upon research over time, not a single study.
- Learn to spot false claims. If something sounds too good to be true, it probably is.

Report Problems

Adverse effects with dietary supplements should be reported to FDA as soon as possible. If you experience such an adverse effect, contact or see your health care professional immediately. Both of you are then encouraged to report this problem to FDA. For information on how to do this, go to *www.cfsan.fda.gov/~dms/ds-rept.html.*

Adverse effects can also be reported to the product's manufacturer or distributor through the address or phone number listed on the product's label. Dietary supplement firms are required to forward reports they receive about serious adverse effects to FDA within 15 days.

For a general, nonserious complaint or concern about dietary supplements, contact your local FDA District Office

(*www.cfsan.fda.gov/~dms/district.html*).

This article appears on FDA's Consumer Health Information Web page (*www.fda.gov/consumer*), which features the latest updates on FDA-regulated products. Sign up for free e-mail subscriptions at *www.fda.gov/consumer/ consumerenews.html.*

For More Information

Protect Your Health
Joint FDA/WebMD resource
www.webmd.com/fda

Fortify Your Knowledge About Vitamins
www.fda.gov/consumer/updates/vitamins111907.html

Tips for the Savvy Supplement User: Making Informed Decisions
www.fda.gov/fdac/features/2002/202_supp.html

Overview of Dietary Supplements
www.cfsan.fda.gov/~dms/ds-oview.html#what

Food Labeling and Nutrition
www.cfsan.fda.gov/label.html

Final Rule Promotes Safe Use of Dietary Supplements
www.fda.gov/consumer/updates/dietarysupps062207.html

In: Dietary Supplements: Primer and FDA...   ISBN: 978-1-60741-891-7
Editors: Timothy H. Riley   © 2010 Nova Science Publishers, Inc.

Chapter 4

FINAL RULE PROMOTES SAFE USE OF DIETARY SUPPLEMENTS

U.S. Food and Drug Administration

Some dietary supplements are beneficial when taken appropriately. Calcium supplements may strengthen bones and folic acid lowers the risk of certain birth defects. But some supplements pose health risks. They may contain harmful ingredients or be improperly manufactured or handled.

On June 22, 2007, FDA announced a final rule establishing current good manufacturing practice requirements (CGMPs) for dietary supplements. In addition, by the end of the year, industry will be required to report all serious dietary supplement adverse events to FDA.

ENSURING QUALITY

Under the final rule, manufacturers are required to evaluate the identity, purity, quality, strength, and composition of dietary supplements.

"The dietary supplement CGMPs should increase consumers' confidence in the quality of the dietary supplement products that they purchase," says Robert E. Brackett, PhD, Director of FDA's Center for Food Safety and Applied Nutrition. "These regulations provide more accountability in the manufacturing process so that consumers can be confident that the products they purchase contain what is on the label."

Inform your doctor about all the supplements you use, especially before surgery.

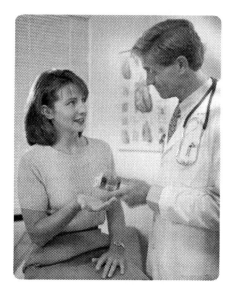

There may be negative interactions associated with some dietary supplements and other medicines you are taking. Consult a health care provider before using any dietary supplement.

The final rule aims to ensure that dietary supplements do NOT have:

- wrong ingredients
- too much or too little of a dietary ingredient
- improper packaging
- improper labeling
- contamination problems due to natural toxins, bacteria, pesticides, glass, lead, or other substances

HOW FDA REGULATES SUPPLEMENTS

The final rule on CGMPs is a critical component of the Dietary Supplement Health and Education Act of 1994 (DSHEA).

Under DSHEA, dietary supplements are regulated like foods. Unlike new drugs, dietary supplements don't have to go through review by FDA for safety and effectiveness or be "approved" before they can be marketed. But manufacturers must provide premarket notice and evidence of safety for any supplements they plan to sell that contain dietary ingredients that were not marketed as dietary supplements before DSHEA was passed—except that the premarket notice is not needed if the new dietary ingredient had previously been used as in ingredient in food.

Manufacturers are responsible for substantiating the safety of dietary ingredients and also for determining that certain structure/function and other claims they make about their products are substantiated by adequate evidence to show that the claims are truthful and not misleading.

FDA evaluates the safety of dietary supplements after they are on the market through research and adverse event monitoring. The agency is responsible for taking action against any unsafe dietary supplement product after it reaches the market.

The final rule on CGMPs gives industry clear expectations for manufacturing, packaging, labeling, and holding dietary supplements. If dietary supplements are found to be contaminated or lacking the appropriate ingredients, FDA will consider those products in violation of the law and will evaluate its enforcement options.

ADVICE FOR CONSUMERS

- **Talk with a health care provider before using a dietary supplement.** This is a good idea, especially for certain population groups. If you are pregnant, nursing a baby, or have a chronic medical condition such as diabetes or heart disease, be sure to consult your doctor or pharmacist before purchasing or taking any supplement.

- **Know that some supplements may interact with prescription and over-the-counter medicines.** Taking a combination of supplements or using these products together with medications (whether prescription or OTC drugs) could produce adverse effects, some of which could be life-threatening. For example, Coumadin (a prescription medicine), ginkgo biloba (an herbal supplement), aspirin (an OTC drug), and vitamin E (a vitamin supplement) can each thin the blood, and taking any of these products together can increase the potential for internal bleeding.

- **Inform your doctor about all the supplements you use, especially before surgery.** Some supplements can have unwanted effects during surgery. You may be asked to stop taking these products at least 2-3 weeks ahead of the procedure to avoid potentially dangerous interactions. These interactions could cause changes in heart rate or blood pressure, increased bleeding, or other problems that could adversely affect the outcome of your surgery.

- **Report adverse effects from the use of dietary supplements to MedWatch.** If you think you have been harmed by a dietary supplement, contact your health provider and report it to FDA's MedWatch program by calling (800) FDA-1088, or visiting *www.fda.gov/medwatch/how.htm*

For more information about the safe use of dietary supplements, visit *www.cfsan.fda.govkvdms/ds-info.html*

To see the final rule on CGMPs for dietary supplements, visit *www.accessdata.fda.gov/scripts/oc/ohrms/dailylist.cfm?yr=2007&mn=6&dy= 25.*

In: Dietary Supplements: Primer and FDA...   ISBN: 978-1-60741-891-7
Editors: Timothy H. Riley   © 2010 Nova Science Publishers, Inc.

Chapter 5

FORTIFY YOUR KNOWLEDGE ABOUT VITAMINS

U.S. Food and Drug Administration

Vitamins are essential nutrients that contribute to a healthy life. Although most people get all the vitamins they need from the foods they eat, millions of people worldwide take supplemental vitamins as part of their health regimen.

WHY BUY VITAMINS?

There are many good reasons to consider taking vitamin supplements, such as over-the-counter multivitamins. According to the American Academy of Family Physicians (AAFP), a doctor may recommend that you take them:

- for certain health problems
- if you eat a vegetarian or vegan diet
- if you are pregnant or breastfeeding

VITAMIN FACTS

Your body uses vitamins for a variety of biological processes, including growth, digestion, and nerve function. There are 13 vitamins that the body absolutely needs: vitamins A, C, D, E, K, and the B vitamins (thiamine, riboflavin, niacin, pantothenic acid, biotin, vitamin B-6, vitamin B-12 and folate). AAFP cites two categories of vitamins.

- **Water-soluble vitamins** are easily absorbed by the body, which doesn't store large amounts. The kidneys remove those vitamins that are not needed.

- **Fat-soluble vitamins** are absorbed into the body with the use of bile acids, which are fluids used to absorb fat. The body stores these for use as needed.

DEVELOP A VITAMIN STRATEGY

It is important for consumers to have an overall strategy for how they will achieve adequate vitamin intakes. The 2005 Dietary Guidelines forAmericans advises that nutrient needs be met primarily through consuming foods, with supplementation suggested for certain sensitive populations.

These guidelines, published by the Department of Health and Human Services and the U.S. Department ofAgriculture (USDA), provide science-based advice to promote health and to reduce risk for chronic diseases through diet and physical activity. They form the basis for federal food, nutrition education, and information programs.

Barbara Schneeman, Ph.D., Director of FDA's Office of Nutritional Products, Labeling, and Dietary Supplements, says, "The Guidelines emphasize that supplements may be useful when they fill a specific identified nutrient gap that cannot or is not otherwise being met by the individual's intake of food." She adds, "An important point made in the guidelines is that nutrient supplements are not a substitute for a healthful diet".

SPECIAL NUTRIENT NEEDS

According to the Dietary Guidelines for Americans, many people consume more calories than they need without taking in recommended amounts of a number of nutrients. The Guidelines warn that there are numerous nutrients—including vitamins—for which low dietary intake may be a cause of concern. These nutrients are:

- calcium, potassium, fiber, magnesium, and vitamins A (as carotenoids), C, and E (for adults)
- calcium, potassium, fiber, magnesium, and vitamin E (for children and adolescents)
- vitamin B-12, iron, folic acid, and vitamins E and D (for specific population groups).

"Do not self-diagnose any health condition. Work with your health care providers to determine how best to achieve optimal health."

Regarding the use of vitamin supplements, the Dietary guidelines include the following:

- **Consume a variety of nutrientdense foods and beverages** within and among the basic food groups. At the same time, choose foods that limit the intake of saturated and trans fats, cholesterol, added sugars, salt, and alcohol.

- **Meet recommended nutrient intakes within energy needs** by adopting a balanced eating pattern, such as one of those recommended in the USDA Food Guide or the National Institute of Health's Dietary Approaches to Stop Hypertension (DASH) eating plan.

- **If you're over age 50**, consume vitamin B-12 in its crystalline form, which is found in fortified foods or supplements.

- **If you're a woman of childbearing age who may become pregnant**, eat foods high in heme-iron and/ or consume iron-rich plant foods or iron-fortified foods with an iron- absorption enhancer, such as foods high in vitamin C.

- **If you're a woman of childbearing age who may become pregnant or is in the first trimester of pregnancy**, consume adequate synthetic folic acid daily (from fortified foods or supplements) in addition to food forms of folate from a varied diet.

- **If you are an older adult, have dark skin, or are exposed to insufficient ultraviolet band radiation (such as sunlight)**, consume extra vitamin D from vitamin D-fortified foods and/or supplements.

Practice Safety with Dietary Supplements

When it comes to purchasing dietary supplements, Vasilios Frankos, Ph.D., Director of FDA's Division of Dietary Supplement Programs, offers this advice: "Be savvy!"

Today's dietary supplements are not only vitamins and minerals. "They also include other less familiar substances such as herbals, botanicals, amino acids, and enzymes," Frankos says. "Check with your health care providers before combining or substituting them with other foods or medicines." Frankos adds, "Do not self-diagnose any health condition. Work with your health care providers to determine how best to achieve optimal health."

Consider the following tips before buying a dietary supplement:

- Think twice about chasing the latest headline. Sound health advice is generally based on research over time, not a single study touted by the media. Be wary of results claiming a "quick fix" that departs from scientific research and established dietary guidance.
- More may not be better. Some products can be harmful when consumed in high amounts, for a long time, or in combination with certain other substances.
- Learn to spot false claims. If something sounds too good to be true, it probably is. Examples of false claims on product labels include:

Quick and effective "cure-all"
Can treat or cure disease
"Totally safe," "all natural," and has "definitely no side effects"

Other red flags include claims about limited availability, offers of "no-risk, money-back guarantees," and requirements for advance payment.

"Also ask yourself, 'Is the product worth the money?'" Frankos advises. "Resist the pressure to buy a product or treatment on the spot. Some supplement products may be expensive or may not provide the benefit you expect. For example, excessive amounts of water-soluble vitamins, like vitamins C and B, are not used by the body and are eliminated in the urine."

How Vitamins are Regulated

Vitamin products are regulated by FDA as "Dietary Supplements." The law defines dietary supplements, in part, as products taken by mouth that contain a "dietary ingredient" intended to supplement the diet.

Listed in the "dietary ingredient" category are not only vitamins, but minerals, botanicals products, amino acids, and substances such as enzymes, microbial probiotics, and metabolites. Dietary supplements can also be extracts or concentrates, and may be found in many forms. The Dietary Supplement Health and Education Act of 1994 requires that all such products be labeled as dietary supplements.

In June 2007, FDA established dietary supplement "current Good Manufacturing Practice" (cGMP) regulations requiring that manufacturers evaluate their products through testing identity, purity, strength, and composition.

Risks of Overdoing It

As is the case with all dietary supplements, the decision to use supplemental vitamins should not be taken lightly, says Vasilios Frankos, Ph.D., Director of FDA's Division of Dietary Supplement Programs.

"Vitamins are not dangerous unless you get too much of them," he says. "More is not necessarily better with supplements, especially if you take fat-soluble vitamins." For some vitamins and minerals, the National Academy of Sciences has established upper limits of intake (ULs) that it recommends not be exceeded during any given day. (For more information, visit *www.nap.edu/catalog.php?record_ id= 6432#toc*

Also, the AAFP lists the following side effects that are sometimes associated with taking too much of a vitamin.

Fat-Soluble Vitamins

- **A (retinol, retinal, retinoic acid):** Nausea, vomiting, headache, dizziness, blurred vision, clumsiness, birth defects, liver problems, possible risk of osteoporosis. You may be at greater risk of these effects if you drink high amounts of alcohol or you have liver problems, high cholesterol levels or don't get enough protein.

- **D (calciferol):** Nausea, vomiting, poor appetite, constipation, weakness, weight loss, confusion, heart rhythm problems, deposits of calcium and phosphate in soft tissues.

If you take blood thinners, talk to your doctor before taking vitamin E or vitamin K pills.

WATER-SOLUBLE VITAMINS

- **B-3 (niacin):** flushing, redness of the skin, upset stomach.

- **B-6 (pyridoxine, pyridoxal, and pyridoxamine):** Nerve damage to the limbs, which may cause numbness, trouble walking, and pain.

- **C (ascorbic acid):** Upset stomach, kidney stones, increased iron absorption.

- **Folic Acid (folate):** High levels may, especially in older adults, hide signs of B-12 deficiency, a condition that can cause nerve damage.

Taking too much of a vitamin can also cause problems with some medical tests or interfere with how some drugs work.

REPORT PROBLEMS

If you believe that you are experiencing an adverse response to taking a vitamin or a dietary supplement, Frankos advises reporting it to your health care provider, as well as to the manufacturer whose name or phone number appears on the label. You can also report directly to FDA through its MedWatch program at 1-800FDA-1088 or online at *www.fda.gov/ medwatch*

Starting December 22, 2007, any serious adverse events reported to a dietary supplement manufacturer must be reported to FDA within 15 days of the manufacturer receiving the adverse event report.

This article appears on FDA's Consumer Health Information Web page (*www.fda.gov/consumer*), which features the latest updates on FDA- regulated products. Sign up for free e-mail subscriptions at *www.fda.gov/ consumer/consumerenews.html.*

FOR MORE INFORMATION

Protect Your Health Joint FDA/WebMD resource *www.webmd.com/fda*

FDA 101: Dietary Supplements *www.fda.gov/consumer/updates/ supplements080408.html*

Dietary Supplements *www.cfsan.fda.govkvdms/ supplmnt.html*

What Dietary Supplements Are You Taking?
www.cfsan.fda.govkvdms/ds-take.html

Dietary Guidelines for Americans, 2005
www.health.gov/dietaryguidelines/ dga2005/document/ default.htm

National Institutes of Health Office of Dietary Supplements
http://dietary-supplements.info.nih.gov/

Dietary Reference Intakes: A Risk Assessment Model for Establishing Upper Intake Levels for Nutrients
www. nap.edu/catalog.php?record_ id= 6432

In: Dietary Supplements: Primer and FDA...   ISBN: 978-1-60741-891-7
Editors: Timothy H. Riley   © 2010 Nova Science Publishers, Inc.

Chapter 6

USING DIETARY SUPPLEMENTS WISELY

U.S. Department of Health and Human Services

Many people take dietary supplements in an effort to be well and stay healthy. With so many dietary supplements available and so many claims made about their health benefits, how can a consumer decide what's safe and effective? This fact sheet provides a general overview of dietary supplements, discusses safety considerations, and suggests sources for additional information.

KEY POINTS

- Federal regulations for dietary supplements are very different from those for prescription and over-the-counter drugs. For example, a dietary supplement manufacturer does not have to prove a product's safety and effectiveness before it is marketed.
- If you are thinking about using a dietary supplement, first get information on it from reliable sources. Keep in mind that dietary supplements may interact with medications or other dietary supplements and may contain ingredients not listed on the label.
- Tell your health care providers about any complementary and alternative practices you use, including dietary supplements. Give them a full picture of what you do to manage your health. This will help ensure coordinated and safe care.

ABOUT DIETARY SUPPLEMENTS

Dietary supplements were defined in a law passed by Congress in 1994 called the Dietary Supplement Health and Education Act (DSHEA). According to DSHEA, a dietary supplement is a product that:

- Is intended to supplement the diet
- Contains one or more dietary ingredients (including vitamins, minerals, herbs or other botanicals, amino acids, and certain other substances) or their constituents
- Is intended to be taken by mouth, in forms such as tablet, capsule, powder, softgel, gelcap, or liquid
- Is labeled as being a dietary supplement.

Herbal supplements are one type of dietary supplement. An herb is a plant or plant part (such as leaves, flowers, or seeds) that is used for its flavor, scent, and/or therapeutic properties. "Botanical" is often used as a synonym for "herb." An herbal supplement may contain a single herb or mixtures of herbs.

Research has shown that some uses of dietary supplements are effective in preventing or treating diseases. For example, scientists have found that folic acid (a vitamin) prevents certain birth defects, and a regimen of vitamins and zinc can slow the progression of the age-related eye disease macular degeneration. Also, calcium and vitamin D supplements can be helpful in preventing and treating bone loss and osteoporosis (thinning of bone tissue).

Research has also produced some promising results suggesting that other dietary supplements may be helpful for other health conditions (e.g., omega-3 fatty acids for coronary disease), but in most cases, additional research is needed before firm conclusions can be drawn.

DIETARY SUPPLEMENT USE IN THE UNITED STATES

A national survey conducted in 2007 found that 17.7 percent of American adults had used "natural products" (i.e., dietary supplements other than vitamins and minerals) in the past 12 months. The most popular products used by adults for health reasons in the past 30 days were fish oil/omega 3/DHA (37.4%), glucosamine (19.9%), echinacea (19.8%), flaxseed oil or pills (15.9%), and ginseng (14.1%). In another, earlier national survey covering all types of dietary supplements, approximately 52 percent of adult respondents said they had used some type of supplement in the last 30 days; the most commonly reported were multivitamins/multiminerals (35 percent), vitamins E and C (12-13 percent), calcium (10 percent), and B-complex vitamins (5 percent).

FEDERAL REGULATION OF DIETARY SUPPLEMENTS

The Federal Government regulates dietary supplements through the U.S. Food and Drug Administration (FDA). The regulations for dietary supplements are not the same as those for prescription or over-the-counter drugs. In general, the regulations for dietary supplements are less strict.

- A manufacturer does not have to prove the safety and effectiveness of a dietary supplement before it is marketed. A manufacturer is permitted to say that a dietary supplement addresses a nutrient deficiency, supports health, or is linked to a particular body function (e.g., immunity), if there is research to support the claim. Such a claim must be followed by the words "This statement has not been evaluated by the Food and Drug Administration. This product is not intended to diagnose, treat, cure, or prevent any disease."
- Manufacturers are expected to follow certain "good manufacturing practices" (GMPs) to ensure that dietary supplements are processed consistently and meet quality standards. Requirements for GMPs went into effect in 2008 for large manufacturers and are being phased in for small manufacturers through 2010.
- Once a dietary supplement is on the market, the FDA monitors safety. If it finds a product to be unsafe, it can take action against the manufacturer and/or distributor, and may issue a warning or require that the product be removed from the marketplace.

Also, once a dietary supplement is on the market, the FDA monitors product information, such as label claims and package inserts. The Federal Trade Commission (FTC) is responsible for regulating product advertising; it requires that all information be truthful and not misleading.

The Federal Government has taken legal action against a number of dietary supplement promoters or Web sites that promote or sell dietary supplements because they have made false or deceptive statements about their products or because marketed products have proven to be unsafe.

SOURCES OF SCIENCE-BASED INFORMATION

It's important to look for reliable sources of information on dietary supplements so you can evaluate the claims that are made about them. The most reliable information on dietary supplements is based on the results of rigorous scientific testing.

To get reliable information on a particular dietary supplement:

- Ask your health care providers. Even if they do not know about a specific dietary supplement, they may be able to access the latest medical guidance about its uses and risks.
- Look for scientific research findings on the dietary supplement. The National Center for Complementary and Alternative Medicine (NCCAM) and the NIH Office of Dietary Supplements, as well as other Federal agencies, have free publications, clearinghouses, and information on their Web sites.

SAFETY CONSIDERATIONS

If you are thinking about or are using a dietary supplement, here are some points to keep in mind.

Tell your health care providers about any complementary and alternative practices you use, including dietary supplements. Give them a full picture of what you do to manage your health. This will help ensure coordinated and safe care. (For tips about talking with your health care providers about CAM, see NCCAM's Time to Talk campaign at nccam.nih.gov/timetotalk/.) It is especially important to talk to your health care provider if you are

- Thinking about replacing your regular medication with one or more dietary supplements.
- Taking any medications (whether prescription or over-the-counter), as some dietary supplements have been found to interact with medications.
- Planning to have surgery. Certain dietary supplements may increase the risk of bleeding or affect the response to anesthesia.

- Pregnant or nursing a baby, or are considering giving a child a dietary supplement. Most dietary supplements have not been tested in pregnant women, nursing mothers, or children.

If you are taking a dietary supplement, **read the label instructions**. Talk to your health care provider if you have any questions, particularly about the best dosage for you to take. If you experience any side effects that concern you, stop taking the dietary supplement, and contact your health care provider. You can also report your experience to the FDA's MedWatch program. Consumer safety reports on dietary supplements are an important source of information for the FDA.

Keep in mind that although many dietary supplements (and some prescription drugs) come from natural sources, **"natural" does not always mean "safe."** For example, the herbs comfrey and kava can cause serious harm to the liver. Also, a manufacturer's use of the term "standardized" (or "verified" or "certified") does not necessarily guarantee product quality or consistency.

Be aware that **an herbal supplement may contain dozens of compounds** and that its active ingredients may not be known. Researchers are studying many of these products in an effort to identify active ingredients and understand their effects in the body. Also consider the possibility that what's on the label may not be what's in the bottle. Analyses of dietary supplements sometimes find differences between labeled and actual ingredients. For example:

- An herbal supplement may not contain the correct plant species.
- The amount of the active ingredient may be lower or higher than the label states. That means you may be taking less—or more—of the dietary supplement than you realize.
- The dietary supplement may be contaminated with other herbs, pesticides, or metals, or even adulterated with unlabeled ingredients such as prescription drugs.

For current information from the Federal Government on the safety of particular dietary supplements, check the "Dietary Supplements: Warnings and Safety Information" section of the FDA Web site at www.cfsan.fda.gov/ ~dms/ds-warn.html or the "Alerts and Advisories" section of the NCCAM Web site at nccam.nih.gov/news/.

DIETARY SUPPLEMENTS RESEARCH AT THE NATIONAL INSTITUTES OF HEALTH

NCCAM, which is part of the National Institutes of Health (NIH), is the Federal Government's lead agency for studying all types of CAM. As part of that role, the Center sponsors a wide array of research to see how dietary supplements might affect the body and tests their use in clinical trials. In fiscal year 2007, NCCAM supported more than 200 research projects studying dietary supplements, including herbs and botanicals.

Also within NIH, the Office of Dietary Supplements (ODS) focuses specifically on dietary supplements, seeking to strengthen knowledge by supporting and evaluating research, disseminating results, and educating the public.

NCCAM and ODS collaborate to fund dietary supplement research centers focused on botanicals, known collectively as the NIH Botanical Research Centers Program. Scientists at the centers conduct basic research and other studies on botanicals and help to select products to be tested in clinical trials. The centers are advancing the scientific base of knowledge about botanicals, making it possible to better evaluate their safety and effectiveness.

NCCAM also sponsors a number of Centers of Excellence for Research on CAM, including centers studying antioxidant therapies, botanicals for autoimmune and inflammatory diseases, grape-derived polyphenols for Alzheimer's disease, and botanicals for pancreatic diseases and for colorectal cancer.

SELECTED REFERENCES

Barnes P.M., Bloom B., Nahin R., (2008) Complementary and alternative medicine use among adults and children: United States, 2007. CDC *National Health Statistics* Report #12..

Dietary Supplement Health and Education Act of 1994. U.S. Food and Drug Administration Web site. Accessed at http://www.fda.gov/opacom/laws/dshea.html on May 12, 2008.

Dietary supplements: background information. Office of Dietary Supplements Web site. Accessed at http://ods.od.nih.gov/factsheets/Dietary Supplements_pf.asp on November 18, 2008.

Dietary supplements: overview. U.S. Food and Drug Administration, Center for Food Safety and Applied Nutrition Web site. Accessed at http://www.cfsan.fda.gov/~dms/supplmnt.html on May 12, 2008.

Natural Medicines Comprehensive Database. Product monographs. Accessed at
    http://www.naturaldatabase.com on May 13, 2008
Radimer K., Bindewald B., Hughes J., et al. (2004). Dietary supplement use by
    US adults: data from the National Health and Nutrition Examination Survey,
    1999-2000. *American Journal of Epidemiology.160(4)*:339-349.

FOR MORE INFORMATION

NCCAM Clearinghouse

The NCCAM Clearinghouse provides information on CAM and NCCAM, including publications and searches of Federal databases of scientific and medical literature. The Clearinghouse does not provide medical advice, treatment recommendations, or referrals to practitioners.

Toll-free in the U.S.: 1-888-644-6226
TTY (for deaf and hard-of-hearing callers): 1-866-464-3615
Web site: nccam.nih.gov
E-mail: info@nccam.nih.gov

Office of Dietary Supplements (ODS)

ODS seeks to strengthen knowledge and understanding of dietary supplements by evaluating scientific information, supporting research, sharing research results, and educating the public. Its resources include publications (such as *What Dietary Supplements Are You Taking*?), fact sheets on a variety of specific supplement ingredients (such as vitamin D and black cohosh), and the International Bibliographic Information on Dietary Supplements (IBIDS) database.

Web site: www.ods.od.nih.gov
E-mail: ods@nih.gov

U.S. Food and Drug Administration (FDA)

The FDA oversees the safety of many products, such as foods, medicines, dietary supplements, medical devices, and cosmetics. Its series of consumer updates includes the publication FDA 101: *Dietary Supplements* (www.fda.gov / consumer/ updates/supplements080408.pdf).

Web site: www.fda.gov Toll-free in the U.S.: 1-888-463-6332

Center for Food Safety and Applied Nutrition (CFSAN)

CFSAN oversees the safety and labeling of supplements, foods, and cosmetics. Online resources for consumers include "Tips for the Savvy Supplement User: Making Informed Decisions and Evaluating Information" and dietary supplement safety alerts.

Web site: www.cfsan.fda.gov

Toll-free in the U.S.: 1–888–723–3366

MedWatch

MedWatch, the FDA's safety information and adverse event reporting program, allows consumers and health care providers to file reports on serious problems suspected with dietary supplements.

Web site: www.fda.gov/medwatch/report/consumer/consumer.htm

Toll-free in the U.S.: 1–888–463–6332

Federal Trade Commission (FTC)

The FTC is the Federal agency charged with protecting the public against unfair and deceptive business practices. A key area of its work is the regulation of advertising (except for prescription drugs and medical devices).

Web site: www.ftc.gov

Toll-free in the U.S.: 1-877-382-4357

PubMed®

A service of the National Library of Medicine (NLM), PubMed contains publication information and (in most cases) brief summaries of articles from scientific and medical journals. CAM on PubMed, developed jointly by NCCAM and NLM, is a subset of the PubMed system and focuses on the topic of CAM.

Web site: www.ncbi.nlm.nih.gov/sites/entrez

CAM on PubMed: nccam.nih.gov/research/camonpubmed/

National Library of Medicine's MedlinePlus and Dietary Supplements Labels Database

To provide resources that help answer health questions, MedlinePlus brings together authoritative information from the National Institutes of Health as well as other Government agencies and health-related organizations.

Web site: www.medlineplus.gov

The Dietary Supplements Labels Database provides information about ingredients in more than 2,000 selected brands of dietary supplements, including vitamins, minerals, herbs or other botanicals, amino acids, and other specialty supplements.

Web site: http://dietarysupplements.nlm.nih.gov/dietary/

ACKNOWLEDGMENTS

NCCAM thanks Jack Killen, M.D., and Carol Pontzer, Ph.D., NCCAM, for their review of this publication. NCCAM also thanks the Office of Dietary Supplements for its review.

This publication is not copyrighted and is in the public domain. Duplication is encouraged.

NCCAM has provided this material for your information. It is not intended to substitute for the medical expertise and advice of your primary health care provider. We encourage you to discuss any decisions about treatment or care with your health care provider. The mention of any product, service, or therapy is not an endorsement by NCCAM.

National Institutes of Health

U.S. Department of Health and Human Services

CHAPTER SOURCES

The following chapters have been previously published:

Chapter 2 - This is an edited, reformatted and augmented version of a United States Government Accountability Office, Report for Congressional Requesters GAO-09-250 dated January, 2009.

Chapter 3 – This is an edited, reformatted and augmented version of a FDA Consumer Health Information / U.S. Food and Drug Administration dated August 4, 2008.

Chapter 4 – This is an edited, reformatted and augmented version of a FDA Consumer Health Information / U.S. Food and Drug Administration dated June 22, 2007.

Chapter 5 – This is an edited, reformatted and augmented version of a FDA Consumer Health Information / U.S. Food and Drug Administration dated February 21, 2009.

INDEX